THE COMPLETE ZERO POINT WEIGHT LOSS COOKBOOK

RD MICHAEL CLARA

COPYRIGHT

Published by

RD Michael Clara

2024 Publication

I

CONTENTS

The table of

INTRODUCTION

In the journey towards achieving and maintaining a healthy weight, many individuals encounter challenges such as complex dietary plans, calorie counting, and restrictive food choices. The Zero Point system presents a transformative approach to weight management.

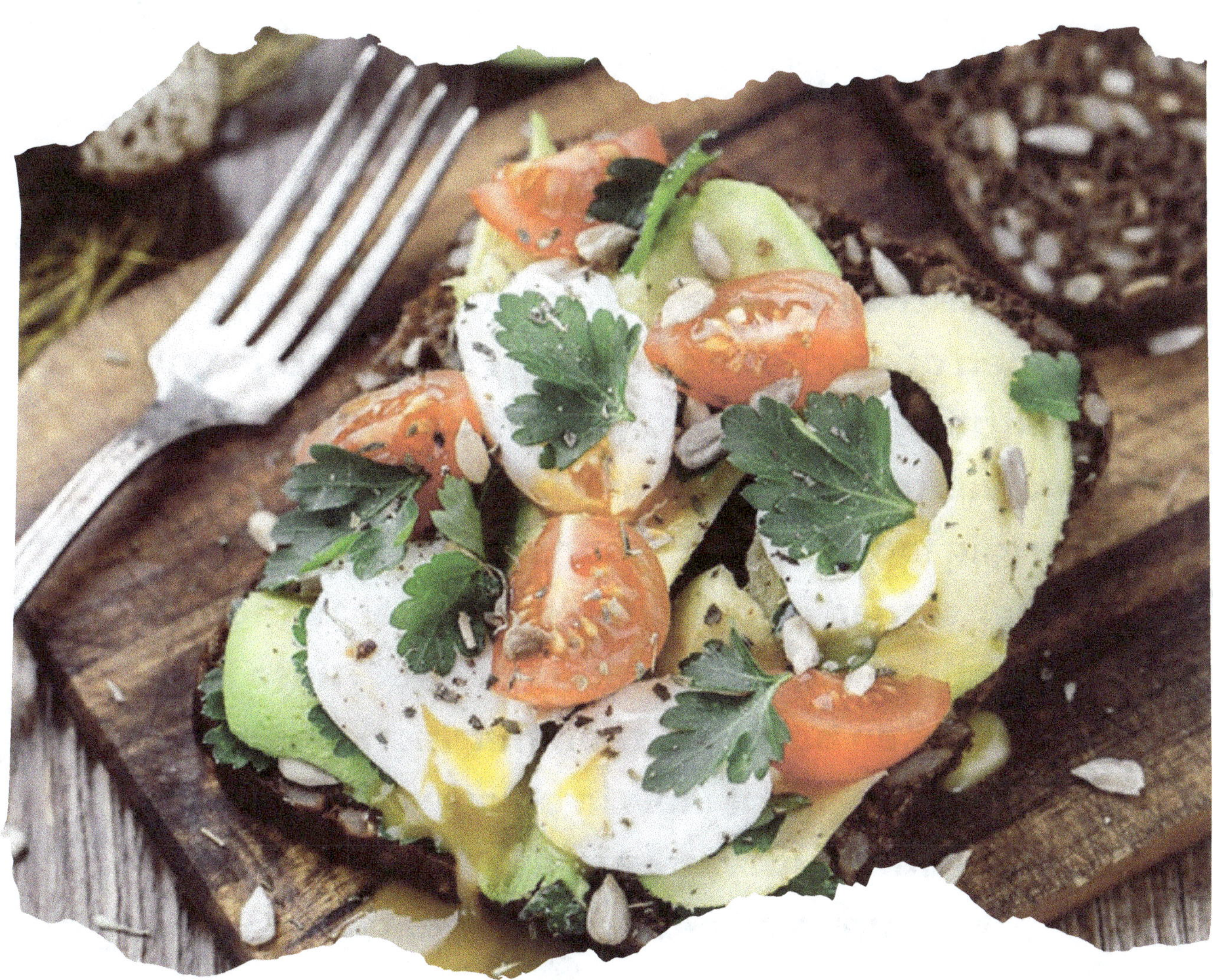

This system is designed to simplify the process by focusing on foods that are not only low in calories but also rich in essential nutrients. By allowing individuals to consume these foods freely without the need for extensive tracking, the Zero Point system empowers people to make healthier choices with ease

Concept of zero point food

The Zero Point system is an innovative concept aimed at promoting healthy eating habits and facilitating sustainable weight loss. The core idea revolves around assigning a "zero point" value to certain foods, which means these items can be consumed in unlimited quantities without impacting your daily caloric intake. These foods are chosen based on their nutritional density, meaning they are low in calories and high in essential nutrients, making them ideal for supporting a healthy lifestyle.

KEY ELEMENTS

Zero Point foods are typically rich in vitamins, minerals, and fiber while being low in calories. This ensures that individuals can enjoy a variety of foods that nourish the body without the worry of overeating.

The system is designed to be straightforward, reducing the complexity often associated with dieting. By eliminating the need to count calories or measure portions for these foods, the Zero Point system makes healthy eating more accessible and less time-consuming.

The selection of Zero Point foods includes a wide range of fruits, vegetables, lean proteins, and whole grains, allowing for a diverse and satisfying diet. This variety not only helps in maintaining interest and enjoyment in meals but also ensures a balanced intake of nutrients.

BENEFITS OF ZERO POINT MEALS

The Zero Point system offers numerous advantages, making it a compelling choice for those looking to lose weight or maintain a healthy lifestyle;

Promotes Healthy Eating Habits: By focusing on whole, unprocessed foods, the Zero Point system encourages the consumption of a balanced diet that supports overall health. This shift helps reduce the intake of added sugars, unhealthy fats, and refined carbohydrates.

Simplifies Meal Planning: With the ability to eat certain foods without counting points, meal planning becomes less stressful and more enjoyable. This simplicity can lead to better adherence to the diet and a higher likelihood of long-term success.

Supports Weight Loss: The inclusion of nutrient-dense, low-calorie foods helps create a calorie deficit, essential for weight loss. By eating more of these foods, individuals can feel full and satisfied, reducing the likelihood of overeating.

Enhances Nutritional Intake: The emphasis on a variety of fruits, vegetables, lean proteins, and whole grains ensures a rich intake of essential nutrients, promoting better health and well-being.

Boosts Motivation and Confidence: The freedom to enjoy a range of foods without constant monitoring can boost confidence and motivation, making the weight loss journey more enjoyable and sustainable.

In conclusion, the Zero Point system represents a revolutionary approach to weight loss and healthy living, making it easier than ever to embrace a balanced diet and achieve personal health goals. By focusing on nutrient-dense, zero point foods, individuals can enjoy a fulfilling and effective weight management journey.

VEGETABLE SOUP

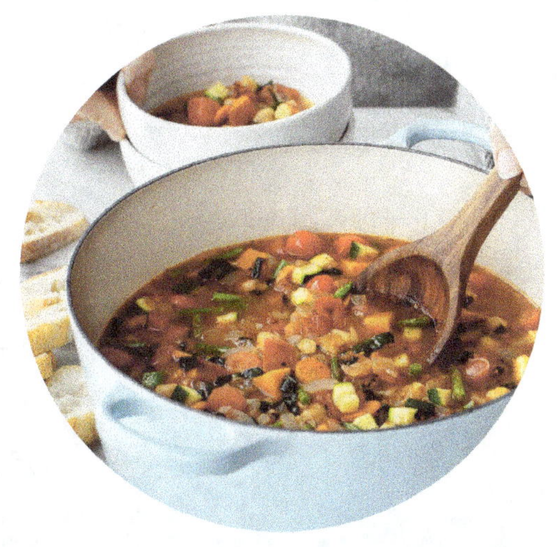

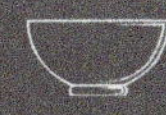 **Preparation Time : 15 min**

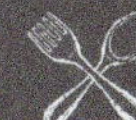 **Total Time : 40 min**

 **Servings : 4**

Ingredients

- 1 large onion, diced
- 2 carrots, peeled and sliced
- 2 celery stalks, sliced
- 2 cloves garlic, minced
- 1 zucchini, diced
- 1 yellow squash, diced
- 1 bell pepper, diced
- 1 cup green beans, trimmed and cut into 1-inch pieces
- 1 can (14.5 oz) diced tomatoes, undrained
- 4 cups vegetable broth
- 1 tsp dried thyme
- 1 tsp dried basil
- 1/2 tsp dried oregano
- Salt and pepper to taste
- 2 cups spinach, chopped
- 1 tbsp olive oil (optional)

Steps for Cooking

- First, prepare the vegetables by dicing the onion, peeling and slicing the carrots, slicing the celery, mincing the garlic, and dicing the zucchini, yellow squash, and bell pepper. Trim and cut the green beans into 1-inch pieces.
- In a large pot, optionally heat the olive oil over medium heat and sauté the onion, carrots, and celery for five minutes. Add the garlic and cook for another minute. Add the zucchini, yellow squash, bell pepper, and green beans, stirring to combine.
- Pour in the diced tomatoes with their juice and the vegetable broth. Season with thyme, basil, oregano, salt, and pepper. Bring the soup to a boil, then reduce the heat and simmer for twenty minutes until the vegetables are tender. Stir in the spinach and cook for an additional five minutes until wilted. Adjust seasoning if necessary and serve hot.

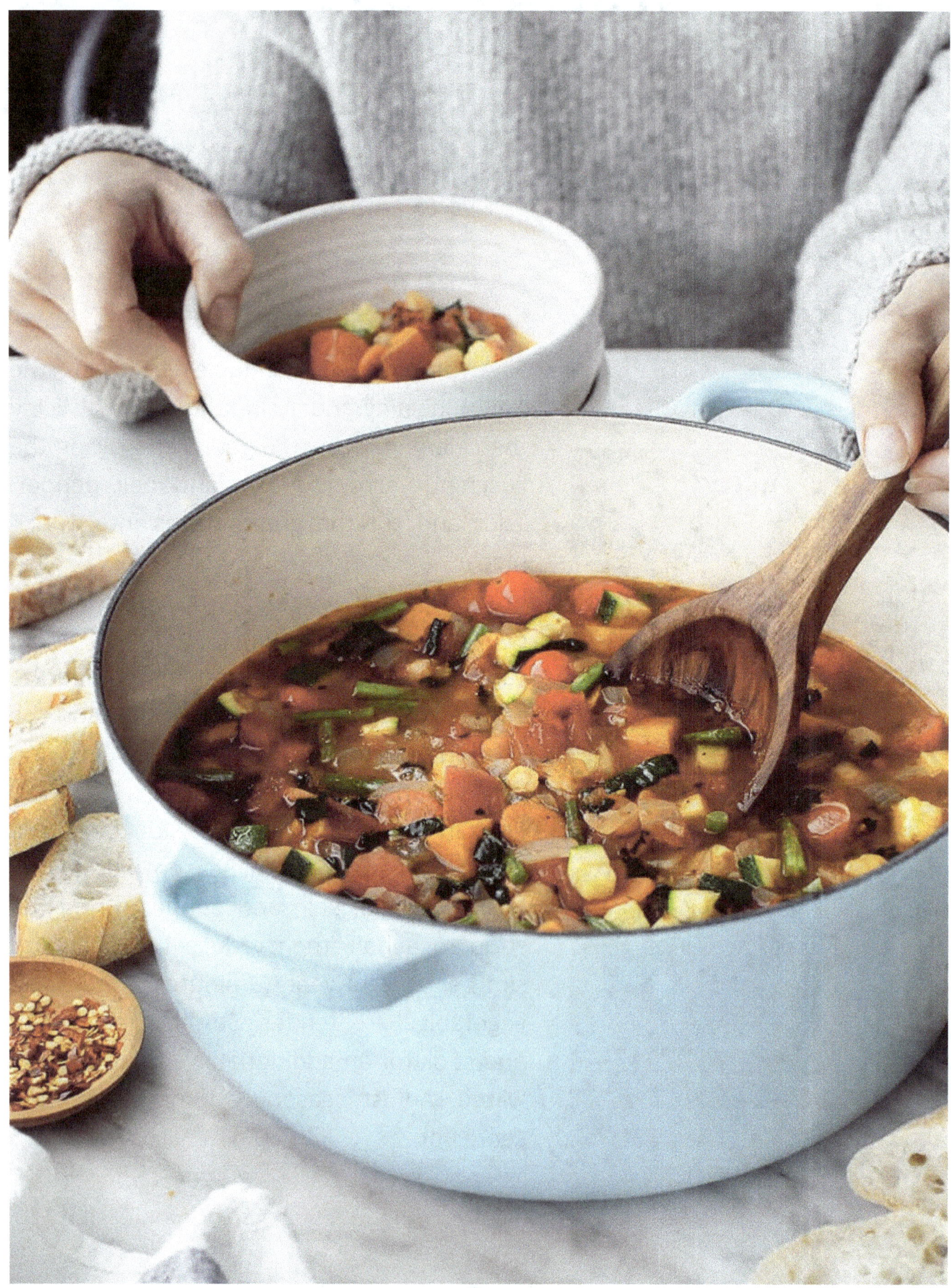

GREEK SALAD

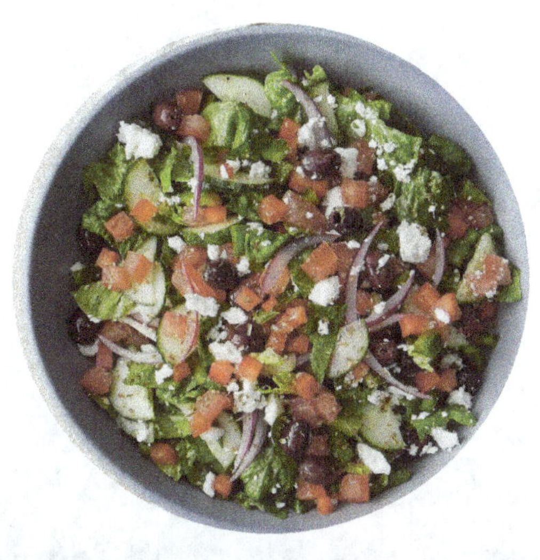

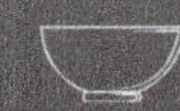 **Preparation Time : 15 min**

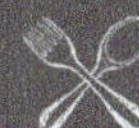 **Total Time : 15 min**

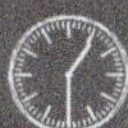 **Servings : 4**

Steps for Cooking

- Begin by preparing all the vegetables. Dice the cucumber and tomatoes, thinly slice the red onion, and dice both the green and red bell peppers.
- In a large bowl, combine the diced cucumber, tomatoes, sliced red onion, and diced bell peppers. Add the Kalamata olives to the bowl.
- In a small bowl, whisk together the olive oil, red wine vinegar, dried oregano, salt, and pepper to make the dressing.
- Pour the dressing over the salad and toss to combine. If using, sprinkle the crumbled feta cheese on top.
- Serve the Greek salad immediately, enjoying it as a refreshing and healthy dish.

Ingredients

- 1 large cucumber, diced
- 4 ripe tomatoes, diced
- 1 red onion, thinly sliced
- 1 green bell pepper, diced
- 1 red bell pepper, diced
- 1/2 cup Kalamata olives, pitted
- 1/2 cup feta cheese, crumbled (optional)
- 2 tablespoons olive oil
- 1 tablespoon red wine vinegar
- 1 teaspoon dried oregano
- Salt and pepper to taste

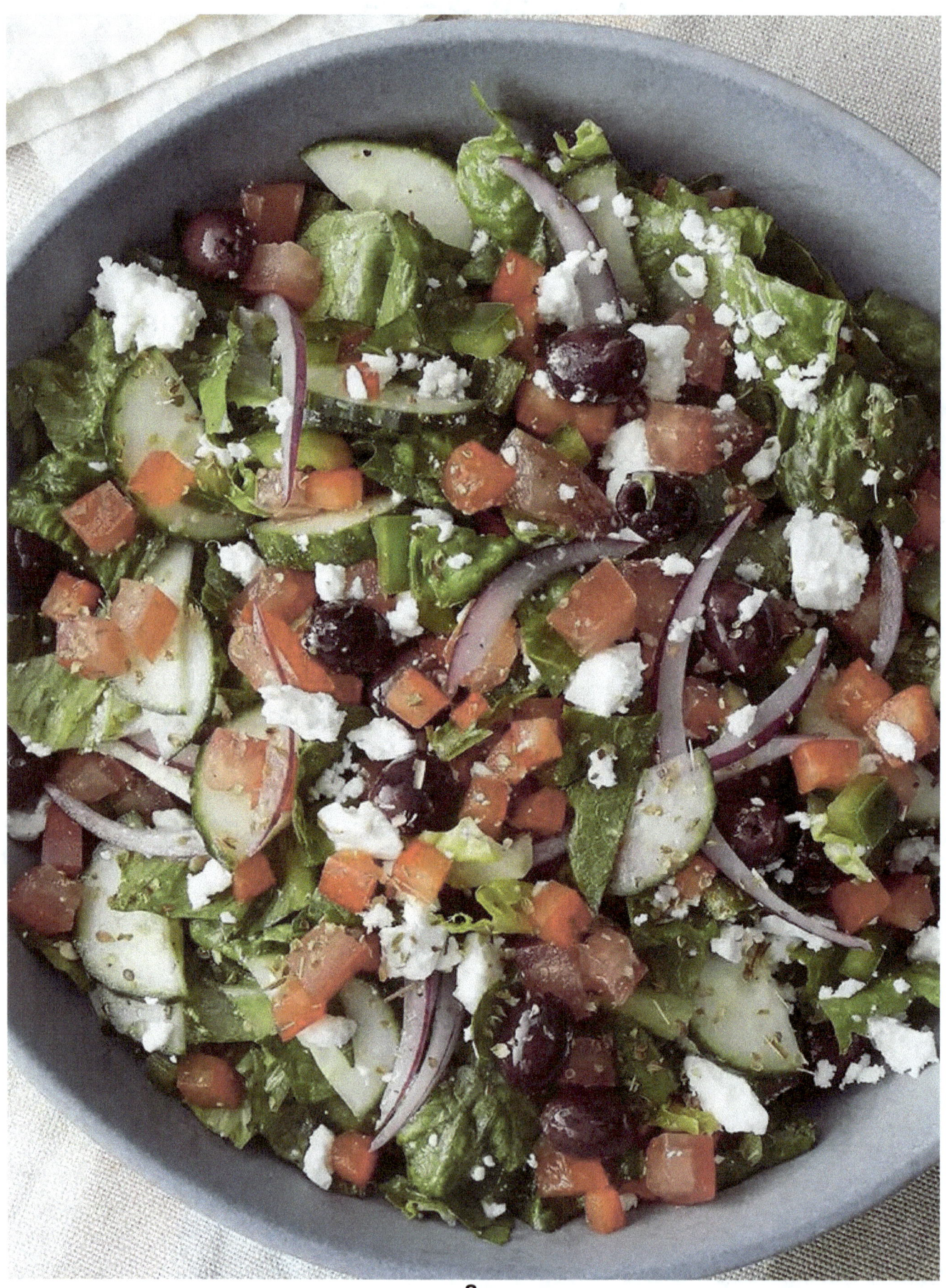

CHICKEN AND VEGGIE STIR-FRY

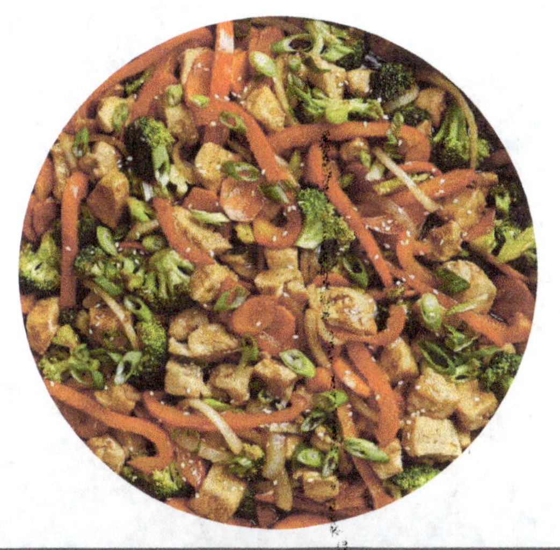

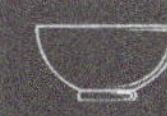
Preparation Time : 15 min

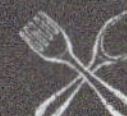
Total Time : 25 min

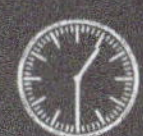
Servings : 4

Ingredients

- 2 boneless, skinless chicken breasts
- 1 red bell pepper, sliced
- 1 yellow bell pepper, sliced
- 1 green bell pepper, sliced
- 1 medium carrot, julienned
- 1 cup broccoli florets
- 1 cup snap peas
- 2 cloves garlic, minced
- 1 tablespoon fresh ginger, minced
- 3 tablespoons low-sodium soy sauce
- 1 tablespoon hoisin sauce (optional)
- 1 tablespoon olive oil or sesame oil
- 1/4 cup water
- 2 green onions, sliced

Steps for Cooking

- First, slice the chicken breasts and all the vegetables. Heat the oil in a large skillet or wok over medium-high heat. Cook the chicken for 5-7 minutes until browned and cooked through. Remove and set aside.
- In the same skillet, sauté the garlic and ginger for about 1 minute. Add the bell peppers, carrot, broccoli, and snap peas, and stir-fry for about 5 minutes until tender-crisp.
- Return the chicken to the skillet, add the soy sauce, hoisin sauce (if using), and water. Stir well and cook for an additional 2-3 minutes until the sauce thickens slightly. Garnish with green onions and sesame seeds if desired, and serve hot.

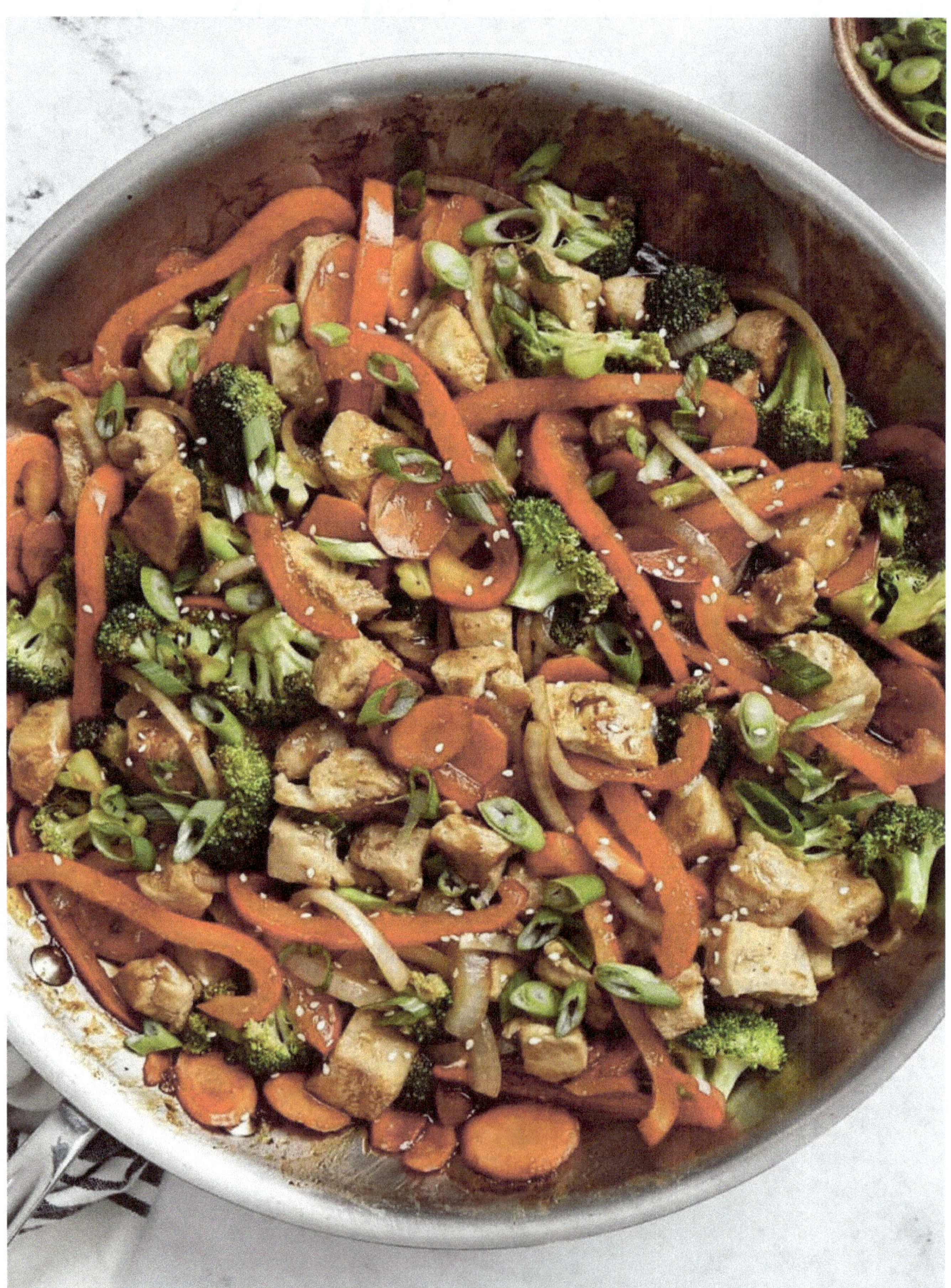

BAKED FISH WITH LEMON & HERB

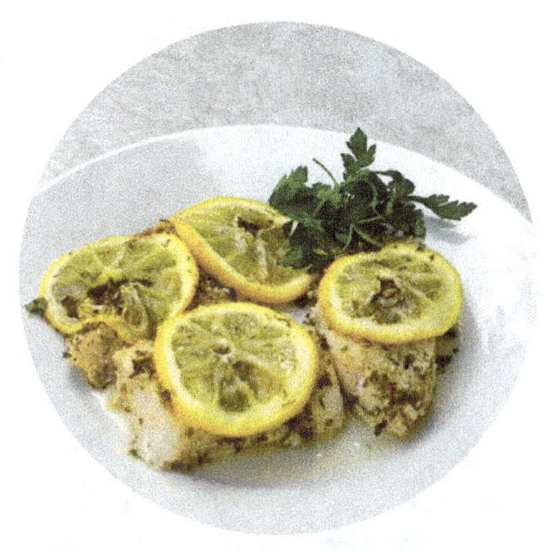

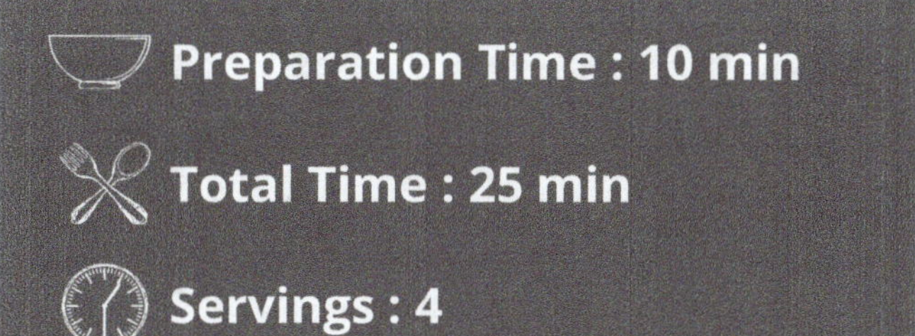

Ingredients

- 4 white fish fillets (such as tilapia or cod)
- 1 lemon, thinly sliced
- 2 tablespoons fresh parsley, chopped
- 2 tablespoons fresh dill, chopped
- 2 cloves garlic, minced
- 1 tablespoon olive oil
- Salt and pepper to taste

Steps for Cooking

- Preheat your oven to 375°F (190°C). Line a baking sheet with parchment paper.
- Place the fish fillets on the prepared baking sheet. Drizzle with olive oil and season with salt and pepper.
- Sprinkle the minced garlic, chopped parsley, and dill evenly over the fish fillets. Arrange the lemon slices on top of the fillets.
- Bake in the preheated oven for 15-20 minutes, or until the fish is cooked through and flakes easily with a fork.
- Serve the baked fish hot, garnished with additional fresh herbs if desired. Enjoy your healthy and flavorful meal!

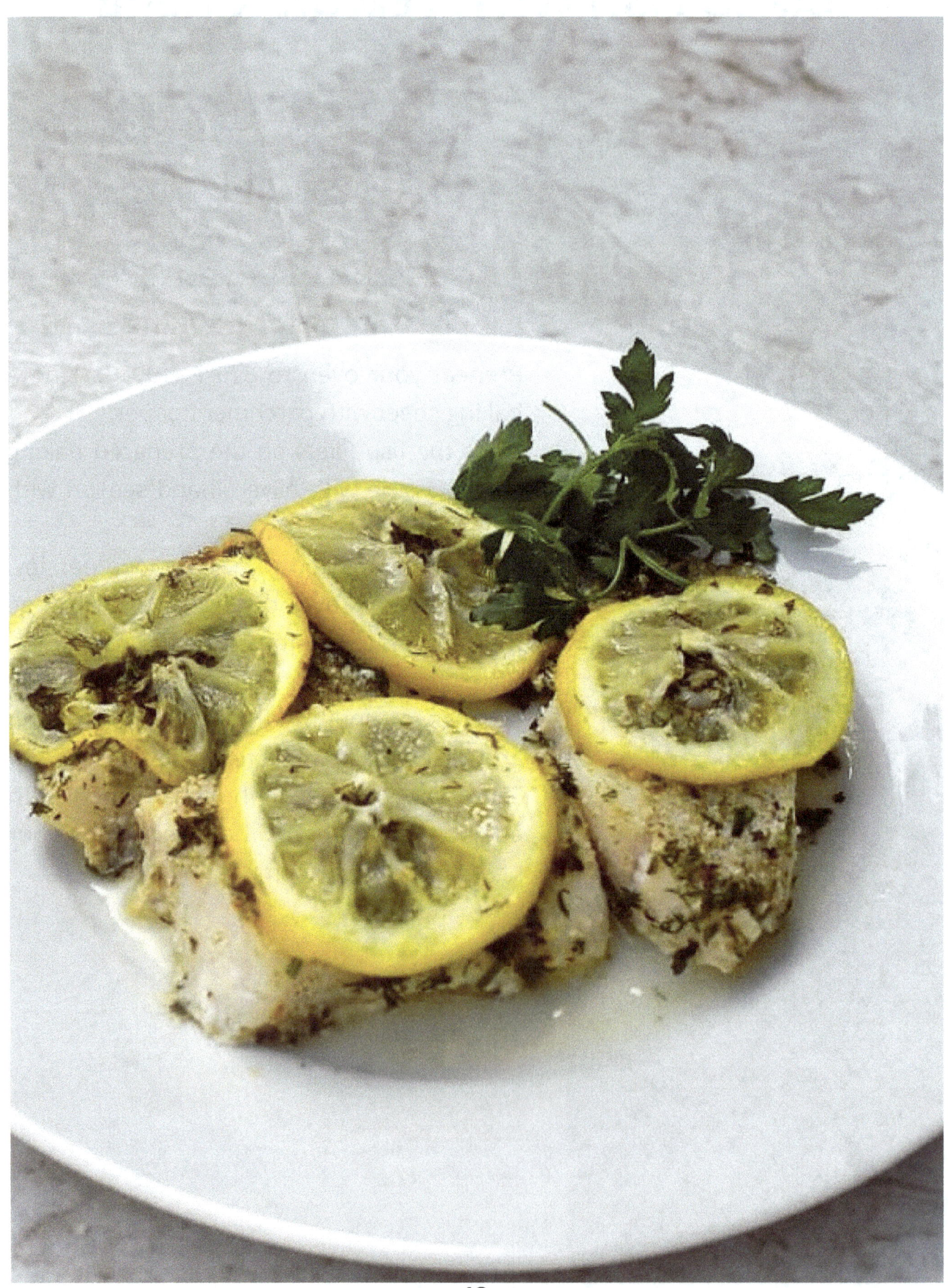

STUFFED BELL PEPPERS

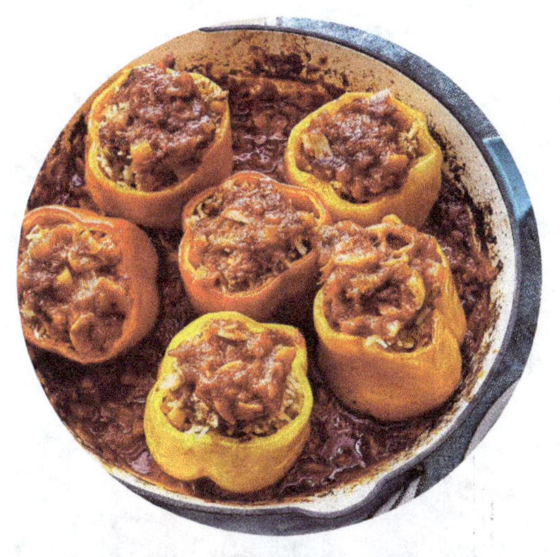

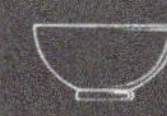 **Preparation Time : 15 min**

 **Total Time : 45 min**

 **Servings : 4**

Ingredients

- 4 large bell peppers (any color)
- 1 lb ground turkey or chicken
- 1 small onion, diced
- 2 cloves garlic, minced
- 1 can (14.5 oz) diced tomatoes, undrained
- 1 cup cooked brown rice or quinoa
- 1 teaspoon dried Italian herbs
- Salt and pepper to taste
- 1 cup shredded mozzarella cheese (optional)

Steps for Cooking

- Preheat your oven to 375°F (190°C). Cut the tops off the bell peppers, remove the seeds and membranes, and place them in a baking dish.
- In a large skillet, cook the ground turkey or chicken over medium heat until browned. Add the diced onion and minced garlic, cooking for about 3 minutes. Stir in the diced tomatoes, cooked rice or quinoa, and Italian herbs. Season with salt and pepper. Let it simmer for 5 minutes.
- Stuff the bell peppers with the mixture, and if desired, top with shredded mozzarella cheese. Cover the dish with foil and bake for 30 minutes. Remove the foil and bake for an additional 5-10 minutes until the peppers are tender and the cheese is melted. Serve hot.

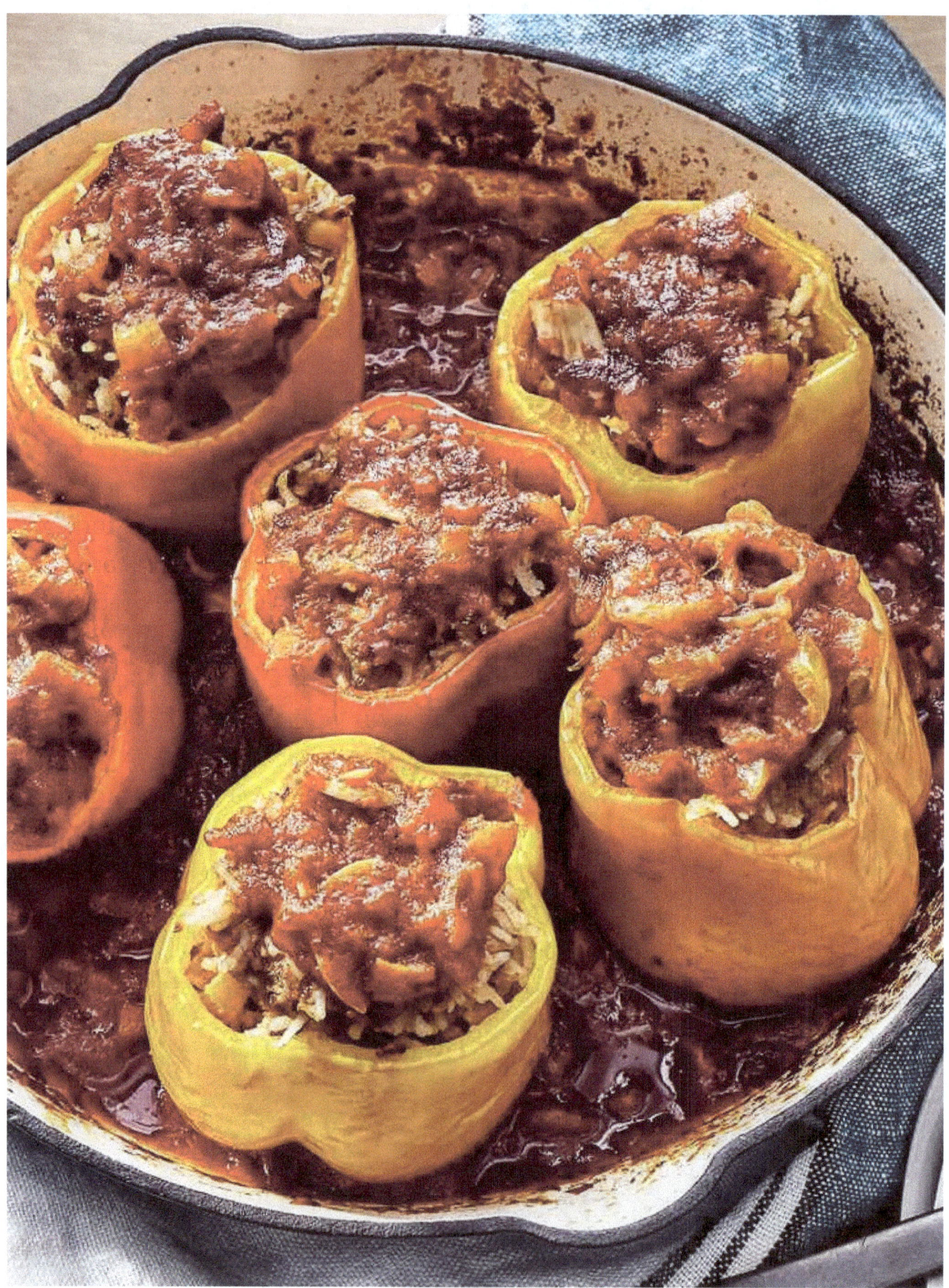

CAULIFLOWER FRIED RICE

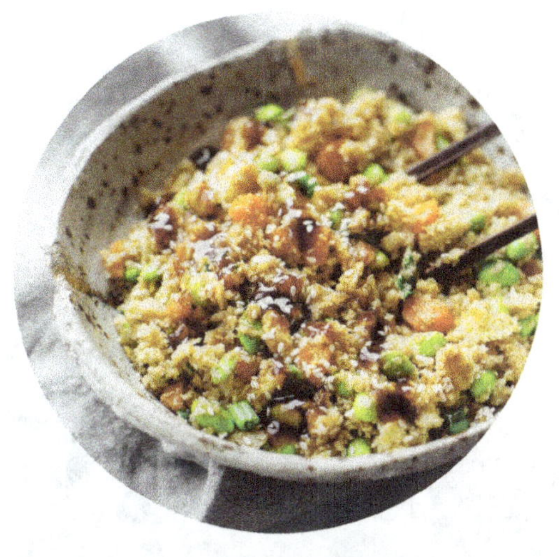

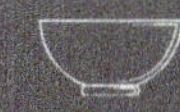
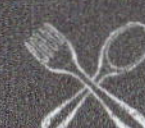
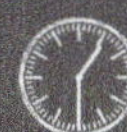

Ingredients

- 1 medium head of cauliflower, grated or 4 cups cauliflower rice
- 2 tablespoons sesame oil or olive oil
- 1 small onion, diced
- 2 cloves garlic, minced
- 1 cup frozen peas and carrots
- 2 large eggs, lightly beaten
- 3 tablespoons low-sodium soy sauce
- 2 green onions, sliced
- Salt and pepper to taste

Steps for Cooking

- First, prepare the cauliflower by grating it or using pre-packaged cauliflower rice.
- In a large skillet or wok, heat one tablespoon of oil over medium-high heat. Add the diced onion and minced garlic, and sauté for about 2 minutes until fragrant.
- Add the frozen peas and carrots to the skillet and cook for another 2-3 minutes until heated through. Push the vegetables to one side of the skillet.
- Pour the beaten eggs into the other side of the skillet and scramble until fully cooked. Mix the eggs with the vegetables.
- Add the remaining tablespoon of oil and the cauliflower rice to the skillet. Stir well to combine and cook for about 5 minutes until the cauliflower is tender.
- Stir in the soy sauce and sliced green onions, cooking for another 2 minutes. Season with salt and pepper to taste.
- Serve the cauliflower fried rice hot, and enjoy a healthy and delicious meal!

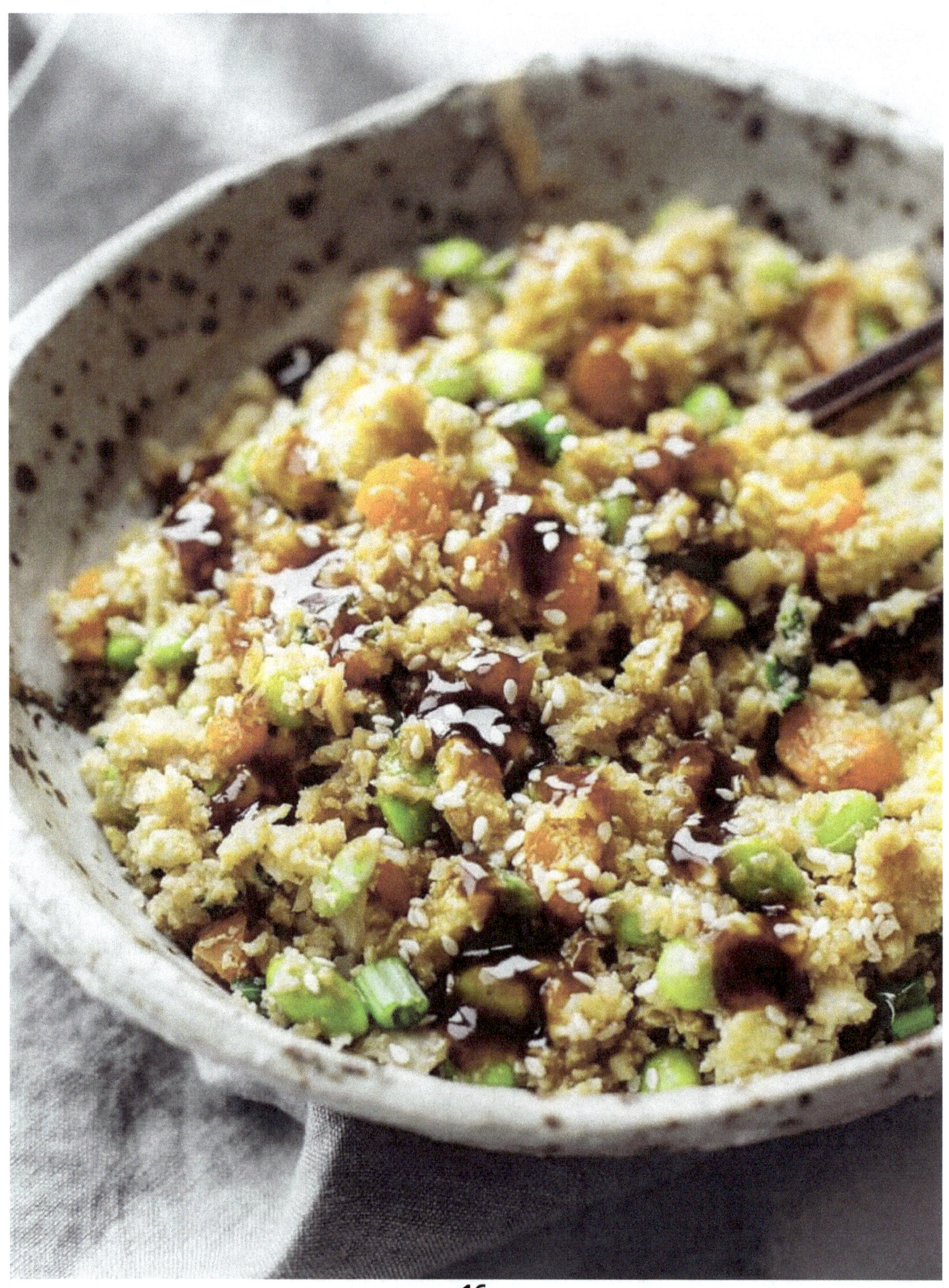

FRUIT SALAD

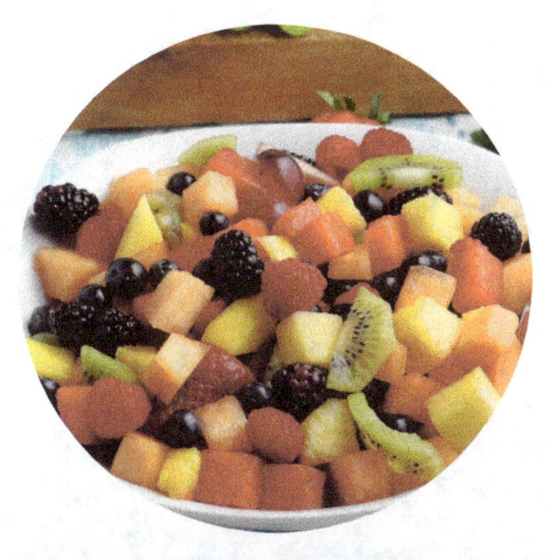

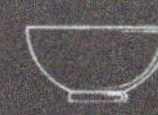 **Preparation Time : 10 min**

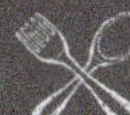 **Total Time : 10 min**

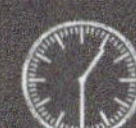 **Servings : 4**

Steps for Cooking

- First, prepare all the fruits by washing, hulling, slicing, and dicing them as needed. In a large mixing bowl, combine the strawberries, blueberries, pineapple, kiwi, grapes, and orange segments.
- If desired, add chopped fresh mint to the bowl for an extra burst of flavor.
- Drizzle the honey or agave syrup (if using) and lime juice over the fruit. Gently toss everything together until well mixed.
- Serve the fruit salad immediately, or chill in the refrigerator for about 30 minutes before serving for an even more refreshing taste. Enjoy your healthy and delicious fruit salad!

Ingredients

- 1 cup strawberries, hulled and sliced
- 1 cup blueberries
- 1 cup pineapple, diced
- 1 cup kiwi, peeled and sliced
- 1 cup grapes, halved
- 1 orange, peeled and segmented
- 2 tablespoons fresh mint, chopped (optional)
- 1 tablespoon honey or agave syrup (optional)
- 1 tablespoon lime juice

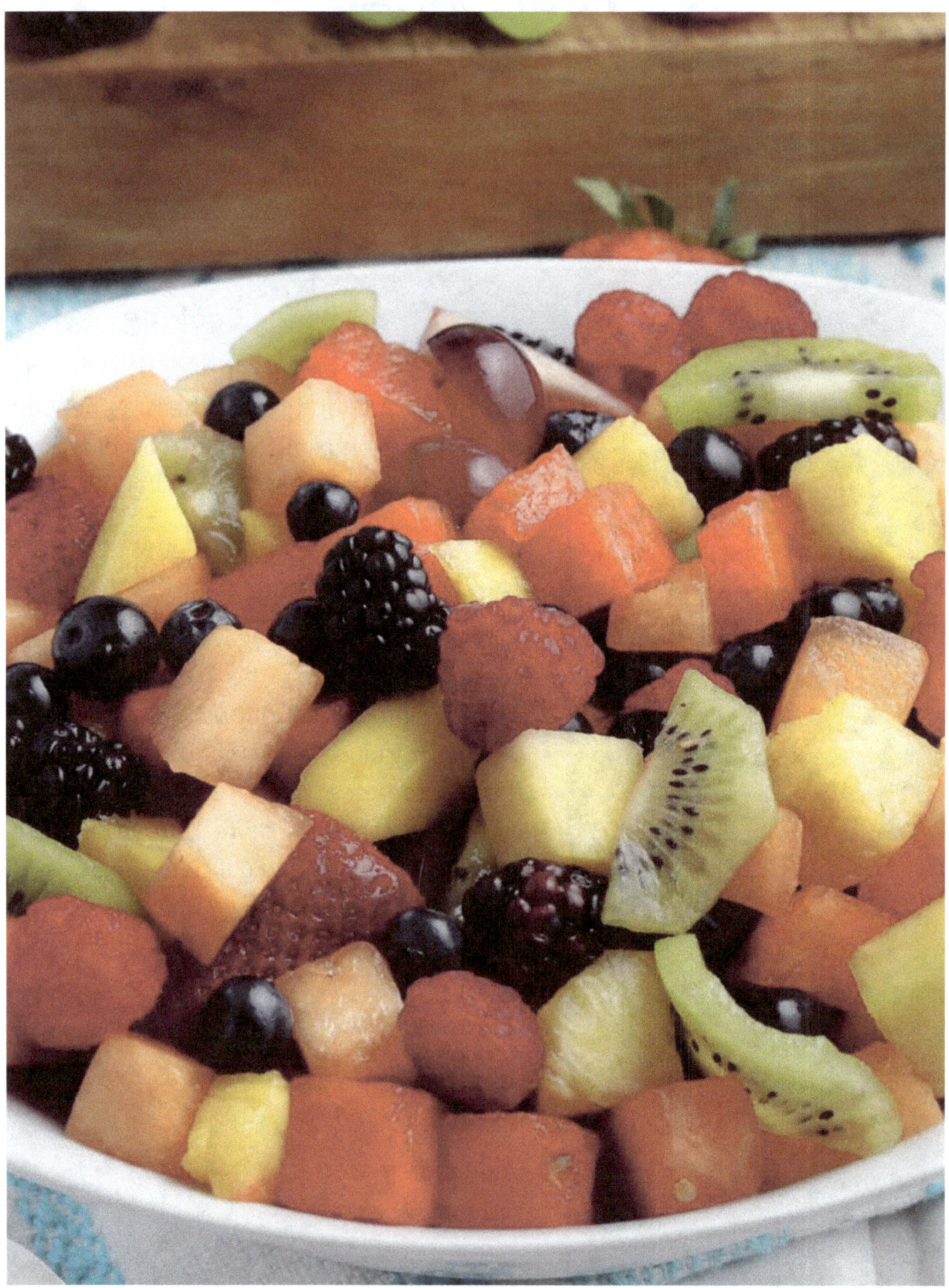

TURKEY LETTUCE WRAPS

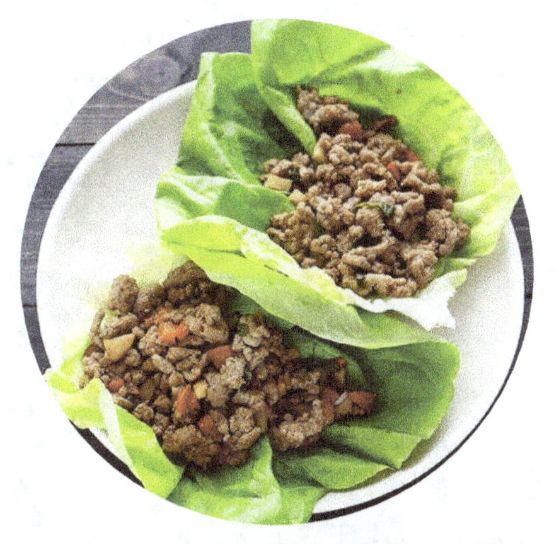

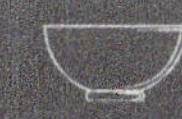 **Preparation Time : 15 min**

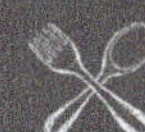 **Total Time : 25 min**

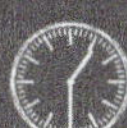 **Servings : 4**

Ingredients

- 1 lb ground turkey
- 1 small onion, diced
- 2 cloves garlic, minced
- 1 bell pepper, diced
- 1 cup water chestnuts, diced
- 3 tablespoons low-sodium soy sauce
- 1 tablespoon hoisin sauce (optional)
- 1 tablespoon rice vinegar
- 1 teaspoon sesame oil
- Salt and pepper to taste
- 1 head of lettuce (butter, iceberg, or romaine), leaves separated
- 2 green onions, sliced (optional)
- 1 tablespoon sesame seeds (optional)

Steps for Cooking

- Start by heating a large skillet over medium-high heat. Add the ground turkey and cook until browned, breaking it up with a spoon as it cooks. This should take about 5-7 minutes.
- Add the diced onion and minced garlic to the skillet, cooking for another 3 minutes until the onion is softened. Stir in the diced bell pepper and water chestnuts, cooking for another 2-3 minutes.
- In a small bowl, whisk together the soy sauce, hoisin sauce (if using), rice vinegar, and sesame oil. Pour this mixture into the skillet with the turkey and vegetables. Stir well to combine and cook for another 2 minutes until everything is heated through. Season with salt and pepper to taste.
- To serve, spoon the turkey mixture into the lettuce leaves. Garnish with sliced green onions and sesame seeds if desired. Enjoy the turkey lettuce wraps immediately as a healthy and delicious meal!

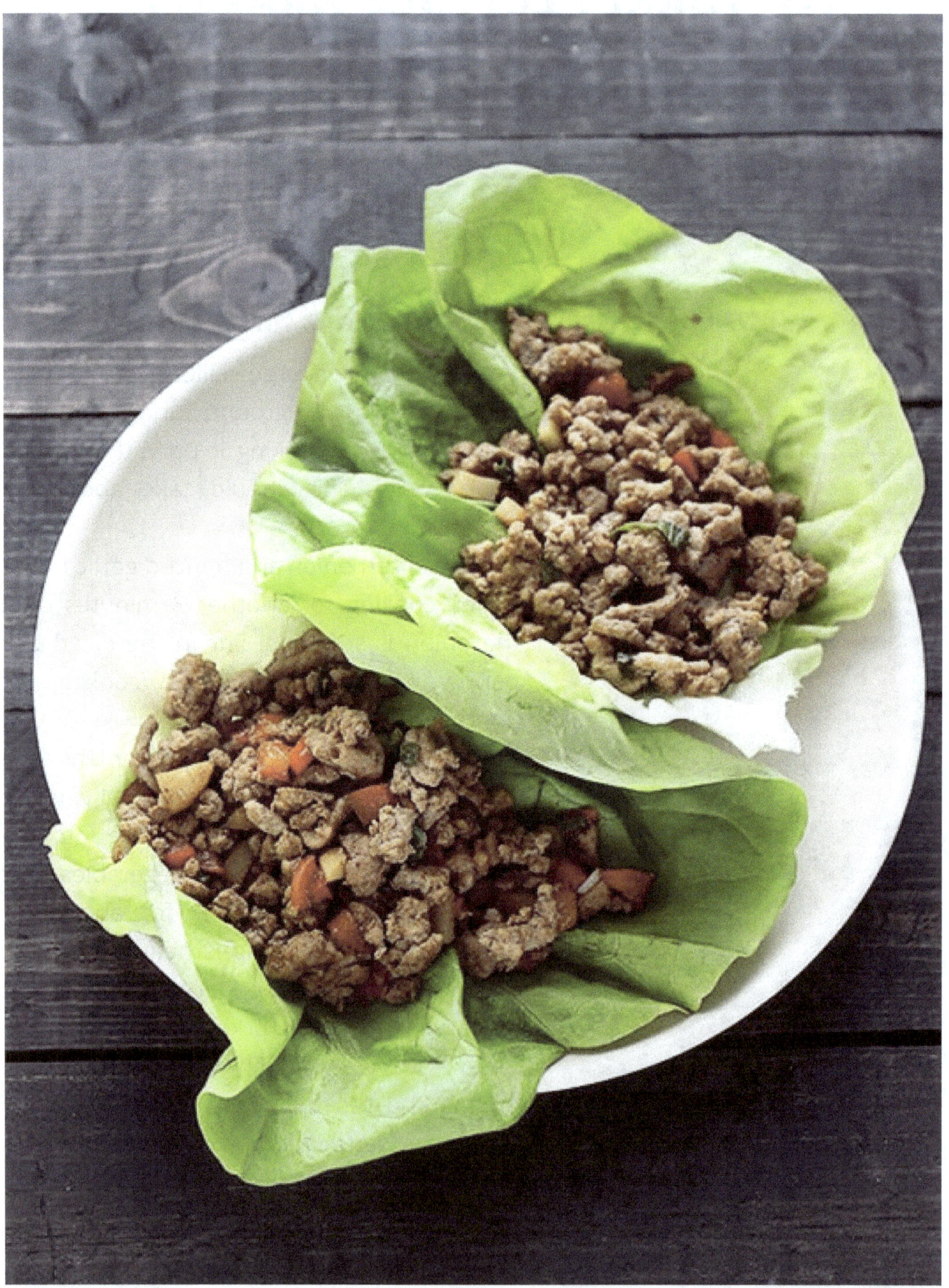

SPAGHETTI SQUASH WITH MARINARA

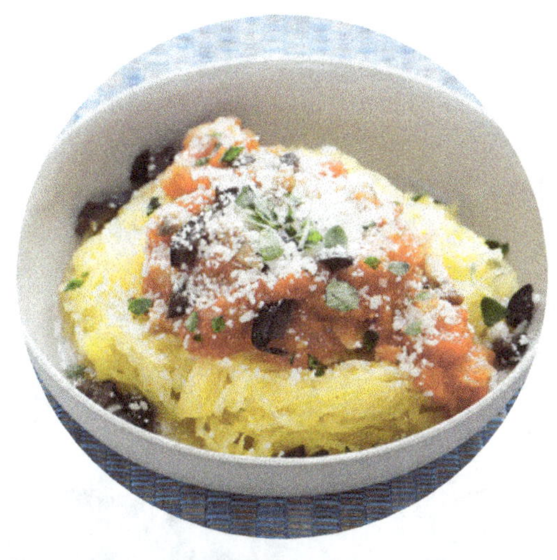

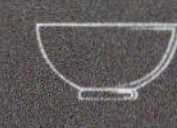
Preparation Time : 10 min

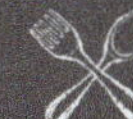
Total Time : 50 min

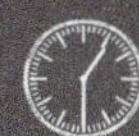
Servings : 4

Ingredients

- 1 large spaghetti squash
- 2 tablespoons olive oil
- Salt and pepper to taste
- 2 cups marinara sauce (store-bought or homemade)
- 1/4 cup grated Parmesan cheese (optional)
- Fresh basil or parsley for garnish (optional)

Steps for Cooking

- Preheat your oven to 400°F (200°C). Carefully cut the spaghetti squash in half lengthwise and scoop out the seeds.
- Drizzle the inside of the squash halves with olive oil and season with salt and pepper. Place the halves cut side down on a baking sheet lined with parchment paper.
- Roast the squash in the preheated oven for 35-40 minutes, or until the flesh is tender and easily pierced with a fork.
- While the squash is roasting, heat the marinara sauce in a saucepan over medium heat until warmed through.
- Once the squash is done, use a fork to scrape out the flesh into spaghetti-like strands. Transfer the strands to a serving dish.
- Pour the warmed marinara sauce over the spaghetti squash strands. If desired, sprinkle with grated Parmesan cheese and garnish with fresh basil or parsley.
- Serve the spaghetti squash with marinara hot, and enjoy a healthy and delicious meal!

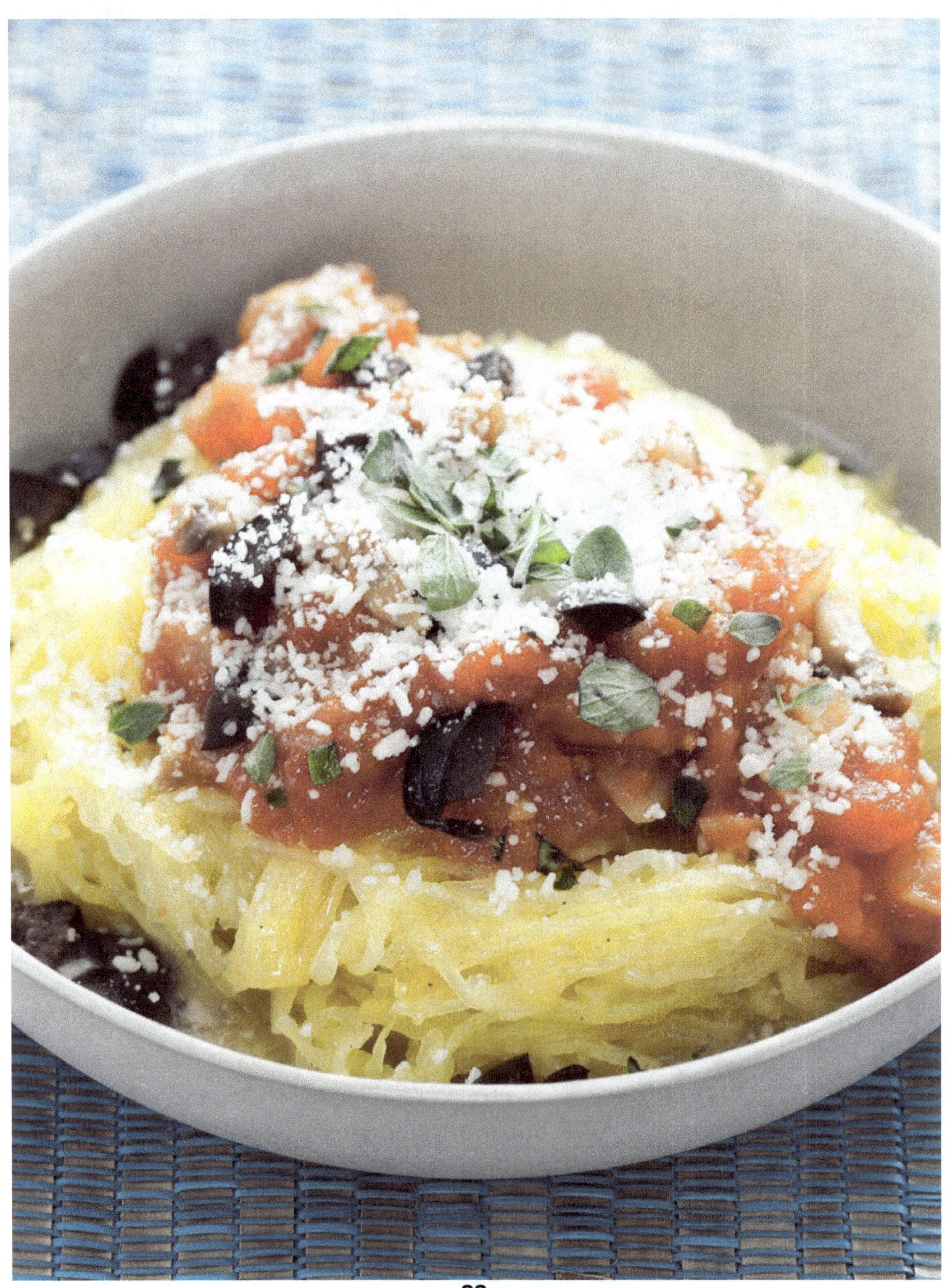

ZUCCHINI NOODLES WITH PESTO

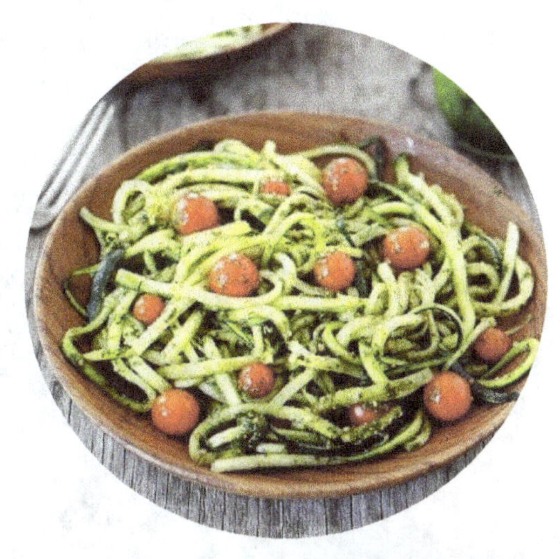

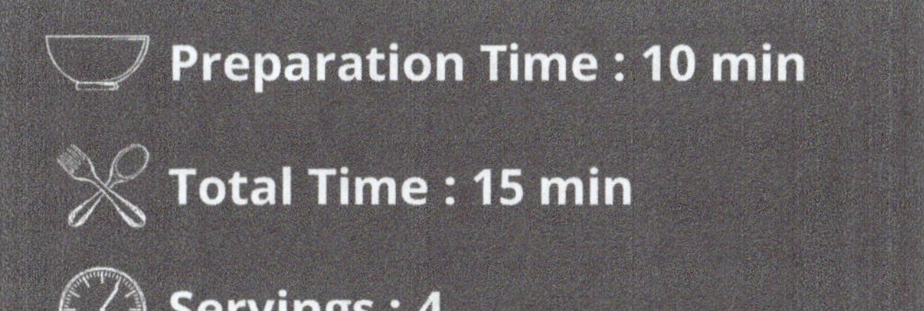

Ingredients

- 4 medium zucchinis, spiralized into noodles
- 1 cup fresh basil leaves
- 1/4 cup pine nuts or walnuts
- 1/4 cup grated Parmesan cheese
- 2 cloves garlic
- 1/4 cup olive oil
- Salt and pepper to taste
- Cherry tomatoes, halved (optional, for garnish)
- Additional grated Parmesan cheese (optional, for garnish)

Steps for Cooking

- First, prepare the zucchini by spiralizing them into noodles. Set the zucchini noodles aside.
- In a food processor, combine the fresh basil leaves, pine nuts or walnuts, grated Parmesan cheese, and garlic. Pulse until the mixture is finely chopped.
- With the food processor running, slowly drizzle in the olive oil until the pesto is smooth and well combined. Season with salt and pepper to taste.
- In a large skillet, heat a small amount of olive oil over medium heat. Add the zucchini noodles and sauté for 2-3 minutes, just until they are tender but still firm (al dente).
- Remove the skillet from heat and toss the zucchini noodles with the prepared pesto until evenly coated.
- If desired, garnish the dish with halved cherry tomatoes and additional grated Parmesan cheese.
- Serve the zucchini noodles with pesto immediately, enjoying a light and flavorful meal!

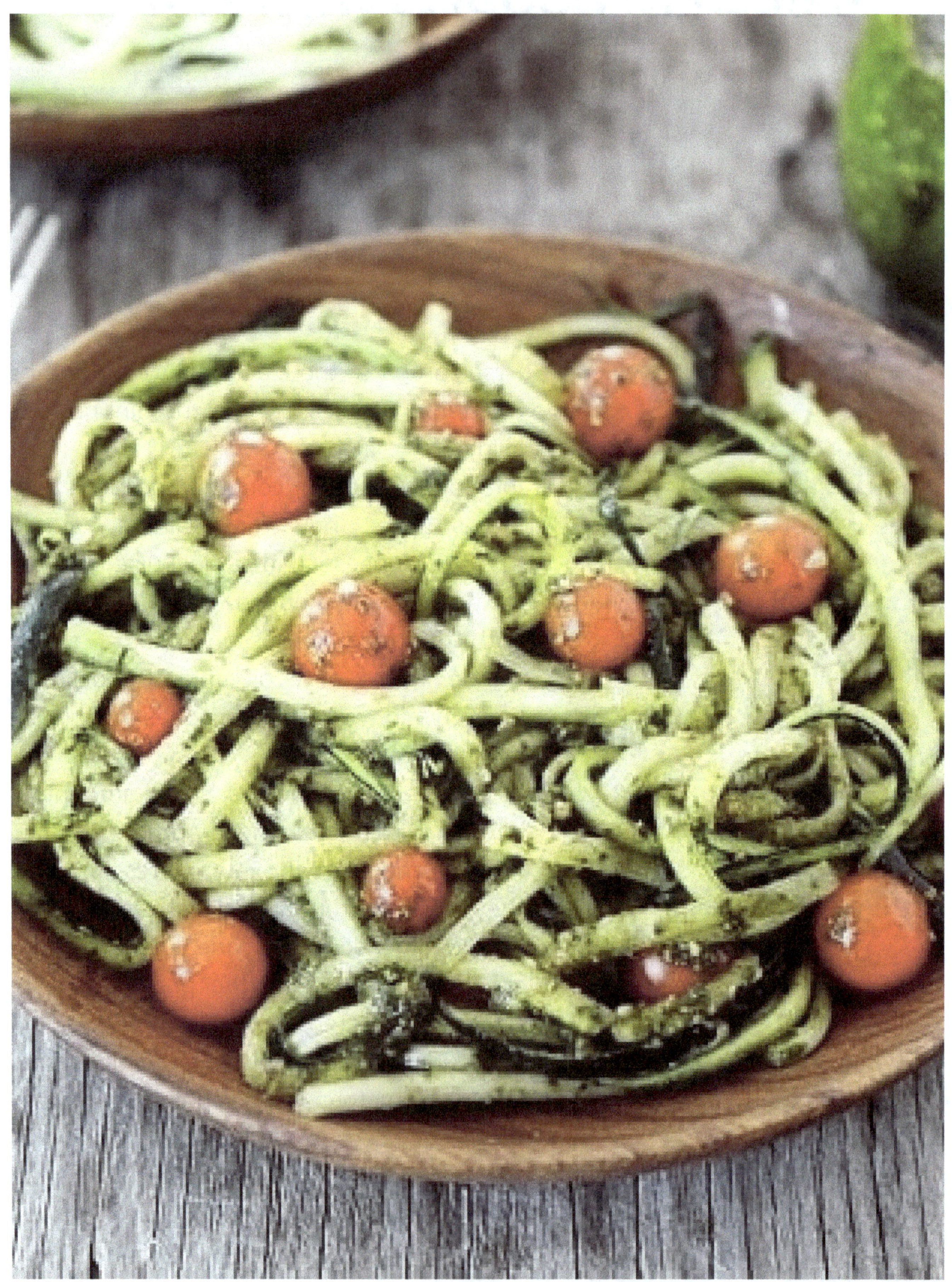

EGG & VEGGIE SCRAMBLE

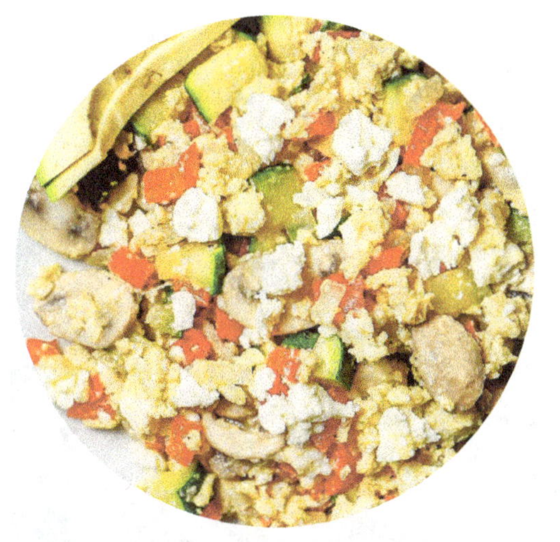

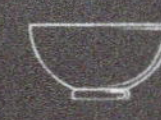
Preparation Time : 10 min

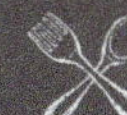
Total Time : 15 min

Servings : 2

Steps for Cooking

- First, whisk the eggs and milk (if using) in a bowl. Season with salt and pepper to taste.
- Heat the olive oil or butter in a large skillet over medium heat. Add the diced onion and bell pepper, and sauté for about 3 minutes until they start to soften.
- Add the diced zucchini, halved cherry tomatoes, and minced garlic to the skillet. Cook for another 2-3 minutes until the vegetables are tender.
- Stir in the chopped spinach and cook until wilted, about 1 minute.
- Pour the beaten eggs over the vegetables in the skillet. Allow the eggs to set slightly, then gently stir and scramble until the eggs are fully cooked.
- Serve the egg and veggie scramble hot, and enjoy a nutritious and delicious meal!

Ingredients

- 4 large eggs
- 1/4 cup milk (optional)
- 1 small onion, diced
- 1 bell pepper, diced
- 1 small zucchini, diced
- 1/2 cup cherry tomatoes, halved
- 1 cup fresh spinach, chopped
- 1 clove garlic, minced
- Salt and pepper to taste
- 1 tablespoon olive oil or butter

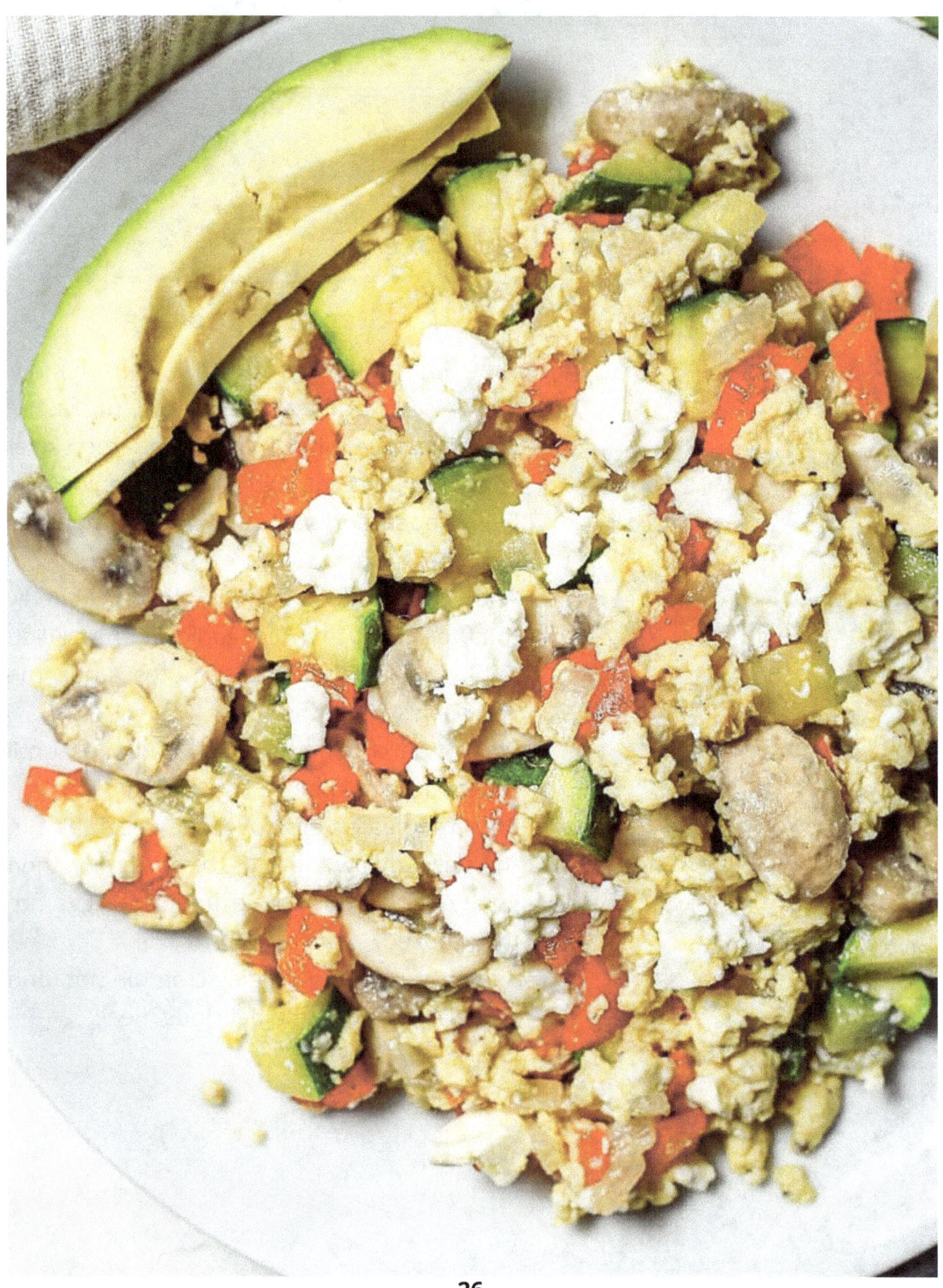

TOMATO BASIL SOUP

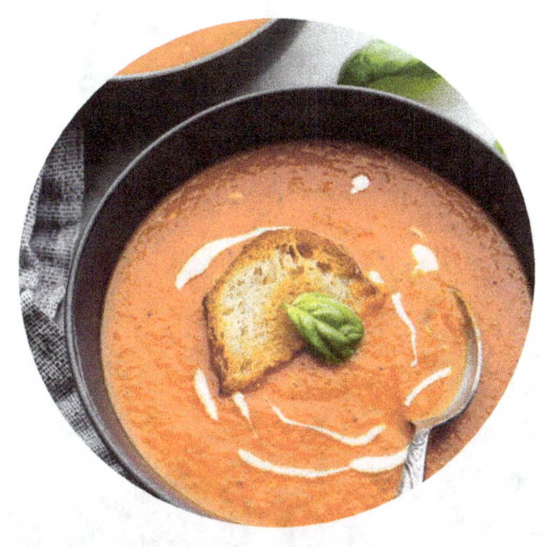

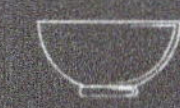 **Preparation Time : 10 min**

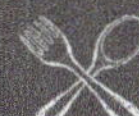 **Total Time : 30 min**

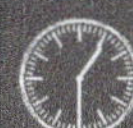 **Servings : 4**

Ingredients

- 1 tablespoon olive oil
- 1 small onion, diced
- 2 cloves garlic, minced
- 4 cups tomatoes, diced (or 2 cans [14.5 oz] diced tomatoes)
- 2 cups vegetable broth
- 1/4 cup fresh basil leaves, chopped
- 1 teaspoon sugar (optional)
- Salt and pepper to taste
- 1/2 cup heavy cream or coconut milk (optional, for creaminess)

Steps for Cooking

- Begin by heating the olive oil in a large pot over medium heat. Add the diced onion and cook for about 5 minutes until softened. Stir in the minced garlic and cook for another minute until fragrant.
- Add the diced tomatoes (with their juices if using canned) and vegetable broth to the pot. Bring to a boil, then reduce the heat and let it simmer for 15 minutes.
- Stir in the chopped fresh basil and sugar (if using). Season with salt and pepper to taste.
- Use an immersion blender to puree the soup until smooth. If you prefer a creamier texture, stir in the heavy cream or coconut milk.
- Serve the tomato basil soup hot, garnished with additional fresh basil if desired. Enjoy your comforting and delicious meal!

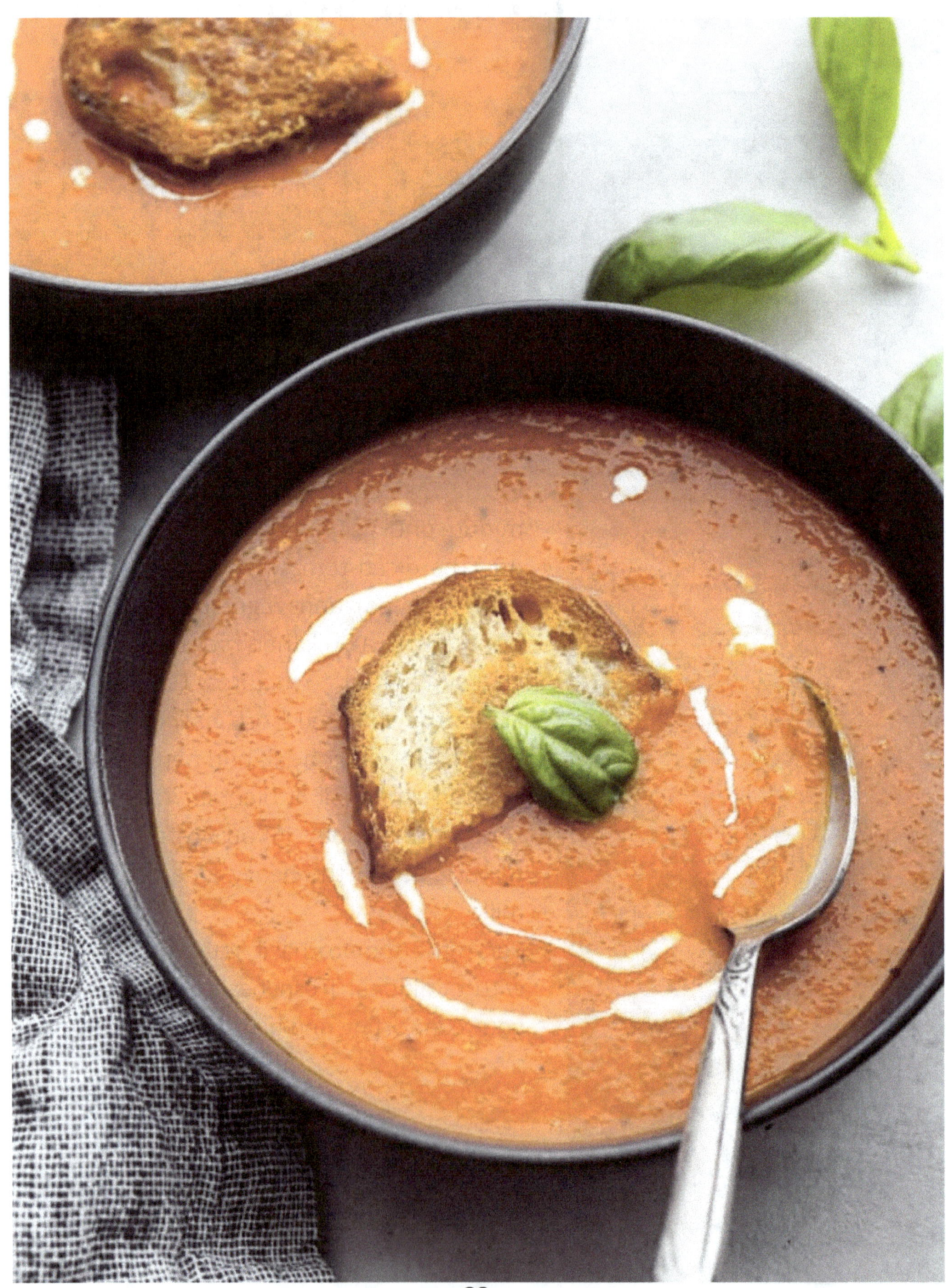

SHRIMP AND AVOCADO SALAD

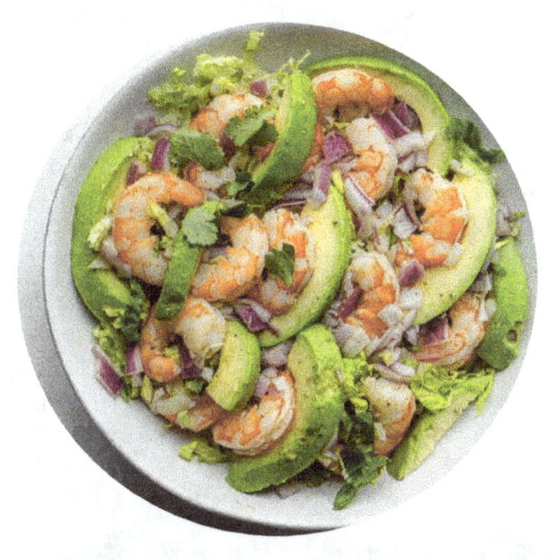

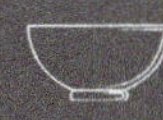
Preparation Time : 15 min

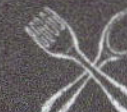
Total Time : 15 min

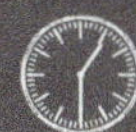
Servings : 4

Ingredients

- 1 lb cooked shrimp, peeled and deveined
- 2 ripe avocados, diced
- 1 cup cherry tomatoes, halved
- 1/2 red onion, thinly sliced
- 1 cucumber, diced
- 1/4 cup fresh cilantro, chopped
- 2 tablespoons olive oil
- 1 tablespoon lime juice
- Salt and pepper to taste

Steps for Cooking

- In a large bowl, combine the cooked shrimp, diced avocados, cherry tomatoes, thinly sliced red onion, diced cucumber, and chopped fresh cilantro.
- In a small bowl, whisk together the olive oil and lime juice. Season with salt and pepper to taste.
- Pour the dressing over the shrimp and avocado mixture, gently tossing to combine and ensure everything is evenly coated.
- Serve the shrimp and avocado salad immediately, enjoying a fresh and flavorful meal!

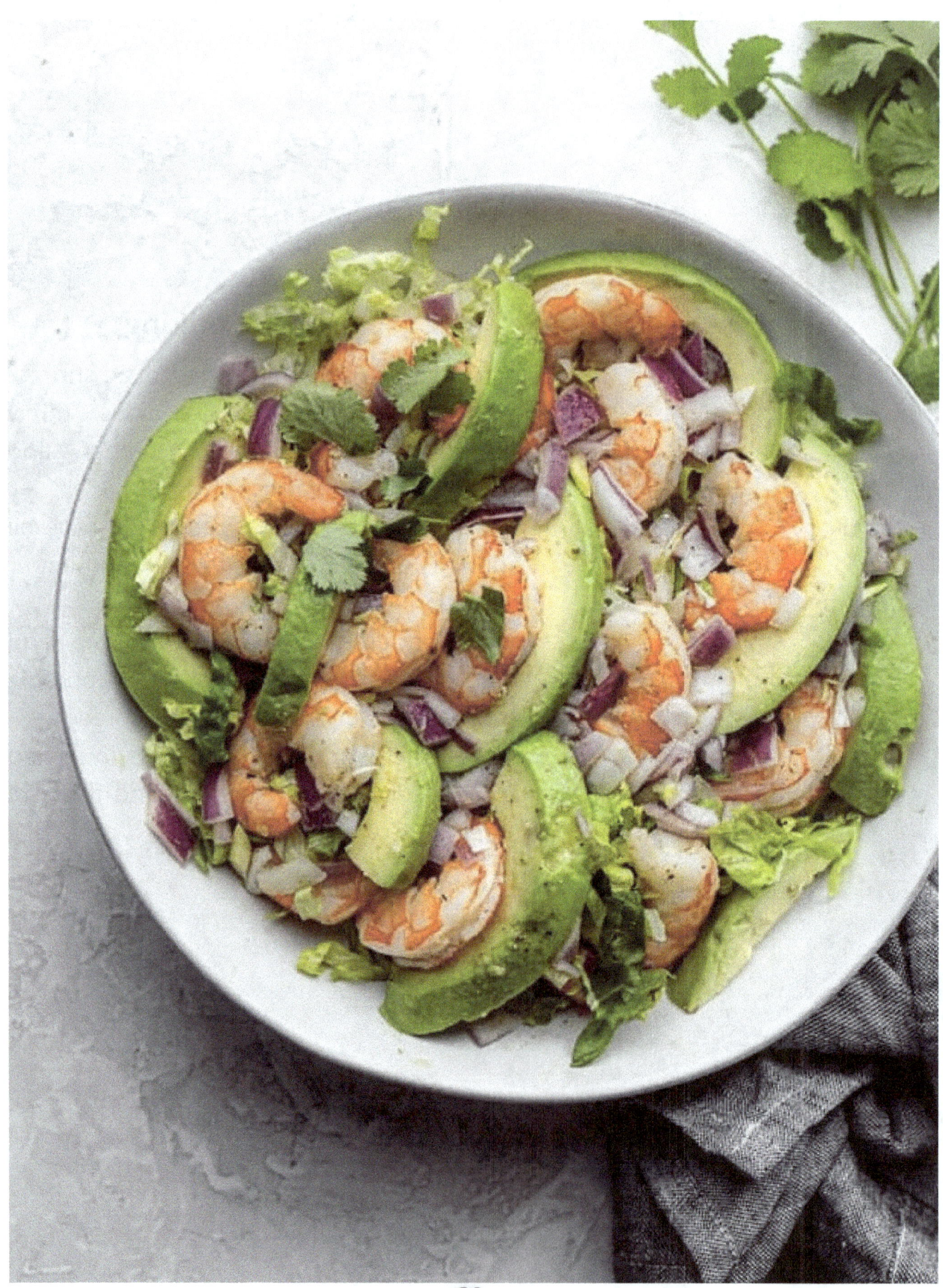

BROILED GRAPEFRUITS

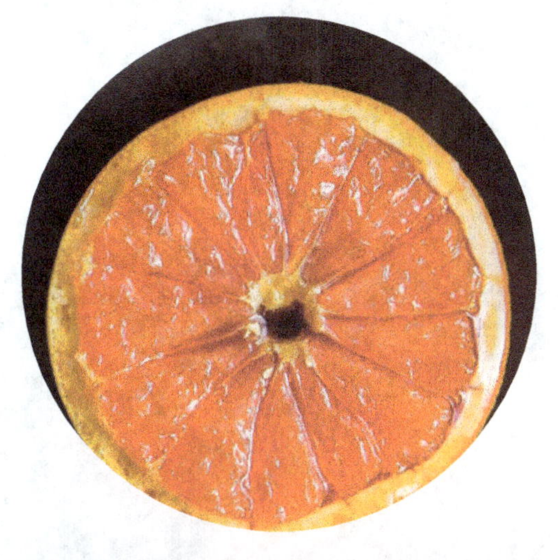

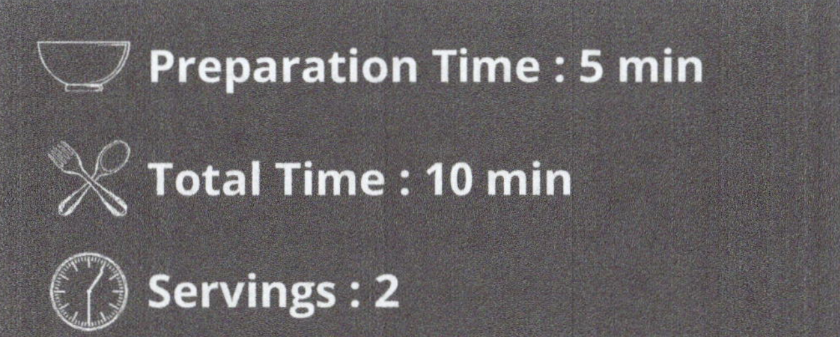

Ingredients

- 1 large grapefruit
- 2 teaspoons brown sugar or honey
- 1/2 teaspoon ground cinnamon
- Optional toppings: fresh mint leaves, yogurt, or granola

Steps for Cooking

- Start by preheating your broiler. Cut the grapefruit in half crosswise.
- Using a small paring knife, loosen the segments of the grapefruit by cutting around the edges and along the membranes.
- Sprinkle each half with 1 teaspoon of brown sugar or honey and a pinch of ground cinnamon.
- Place the grapefruit halves on a baking sheet, cut side up. Broil for 3-5 minutes until the sugar is bubbly and slightly caramelized.
- Remove from the oven and let it cool slightly. If desired, top with fresh mint leaves, a dollop of yogurt, or a sprinkle of granola before serving.
- Enjoy your broiled grapefruit as a delicious and healthy treat!

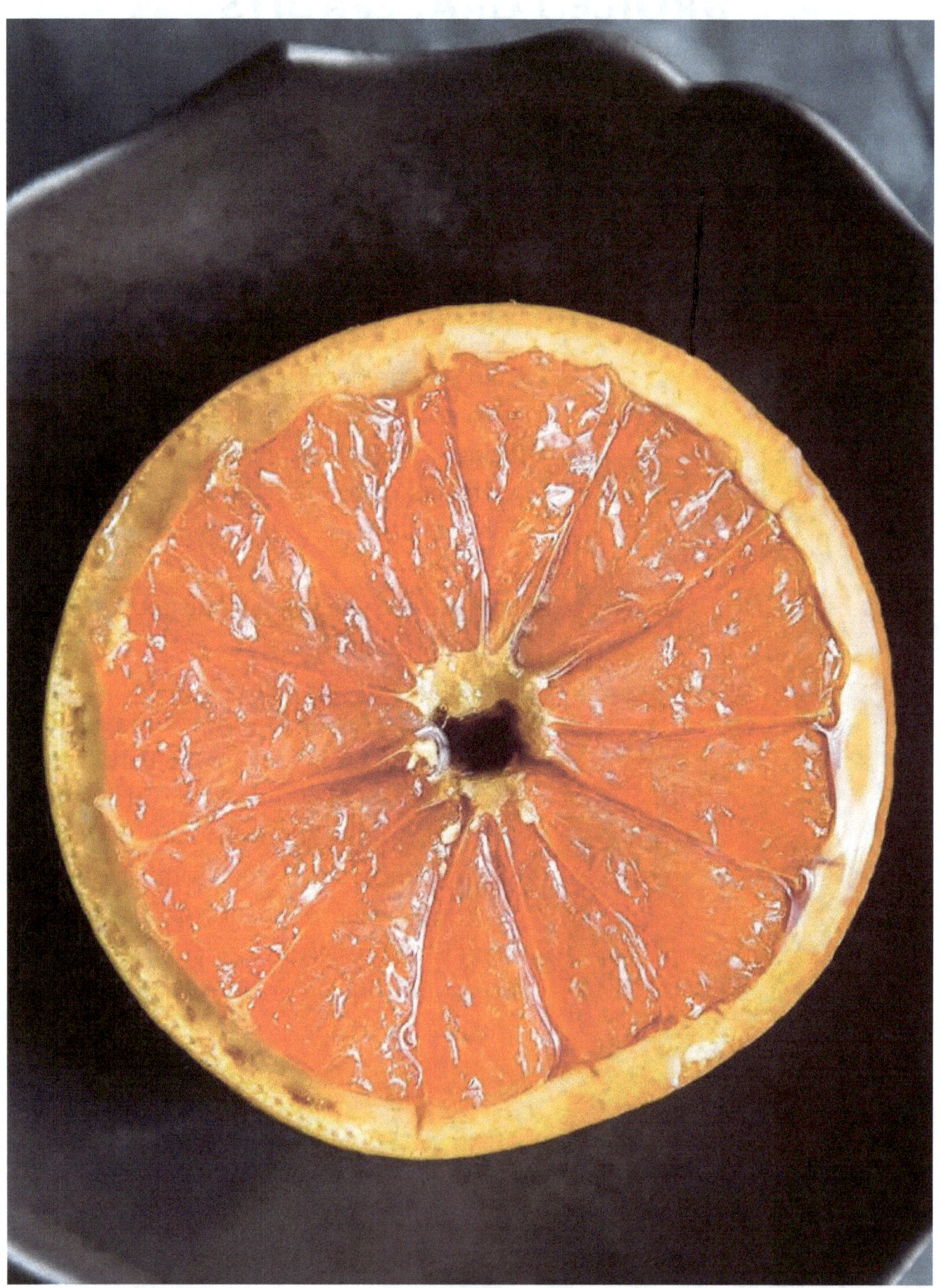

CHICKEN VEGETABLE KABOBS

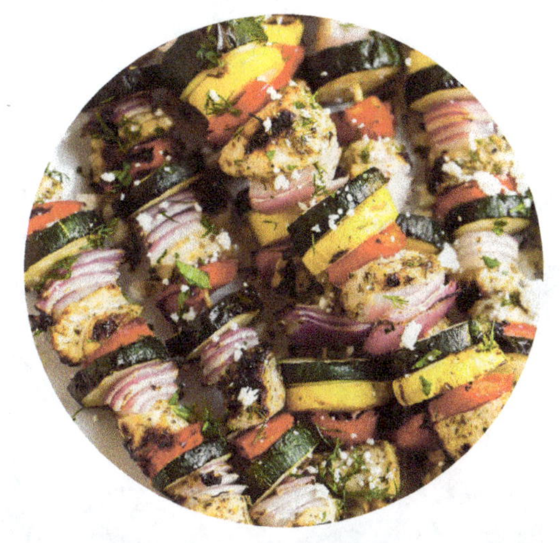

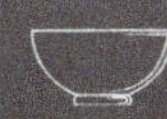 **Preparation Time : 20 min**

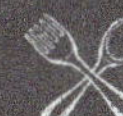 **Total Time : 40 min**

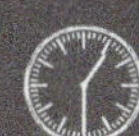 **Servings : 4**

Ingredients

- 1 lb boneless, skinless chicken breasts, cut into 1-inch cubes
- 1 red bell pepper, cut into 1-inch pieces
- 1 yellow bell pepper, cut into 1-inch pieces
- 1 zucchini, sliced into 1/2-inch rounds
- 1 red onion, cut into wedges
- 1/4 cup olive oil
- 2 tablespoons lemon juice
- 2 cloves garlic, minced
- 1 teaspoon dried oregano
- Salt and pepper to taste
- Wooden or metal skewers

Steps for Cooking

- If using wooden skewers, soak them in water for at least 30 minutes to prevent burning.
- In a large bowl, combine the olive oil, lemon juice, minced garlic, dried oregano, salt, and pepper to create the marinade.
- Add the chicken cubes to the marinade, tossing to coat well. Let it marinate for at least 15 minutes.
- Preheat your grill to medium-high heat.
- Thread the marinated chicken, red bell pepper, yellow bell pepper, zucchini, and red onion pieces onto the skewers, alternating between the chicken and vegetables.
- Grill the kabobs for about 10-12 minutes, turning occasionally, until the chicken is fully cooked and the vegetables are tender and slightly charred.
- Remove the kabobs from the grill and let them rest for a few minutes before serving. Enjoy your delicious and healthy chicken vegetable kabobs!

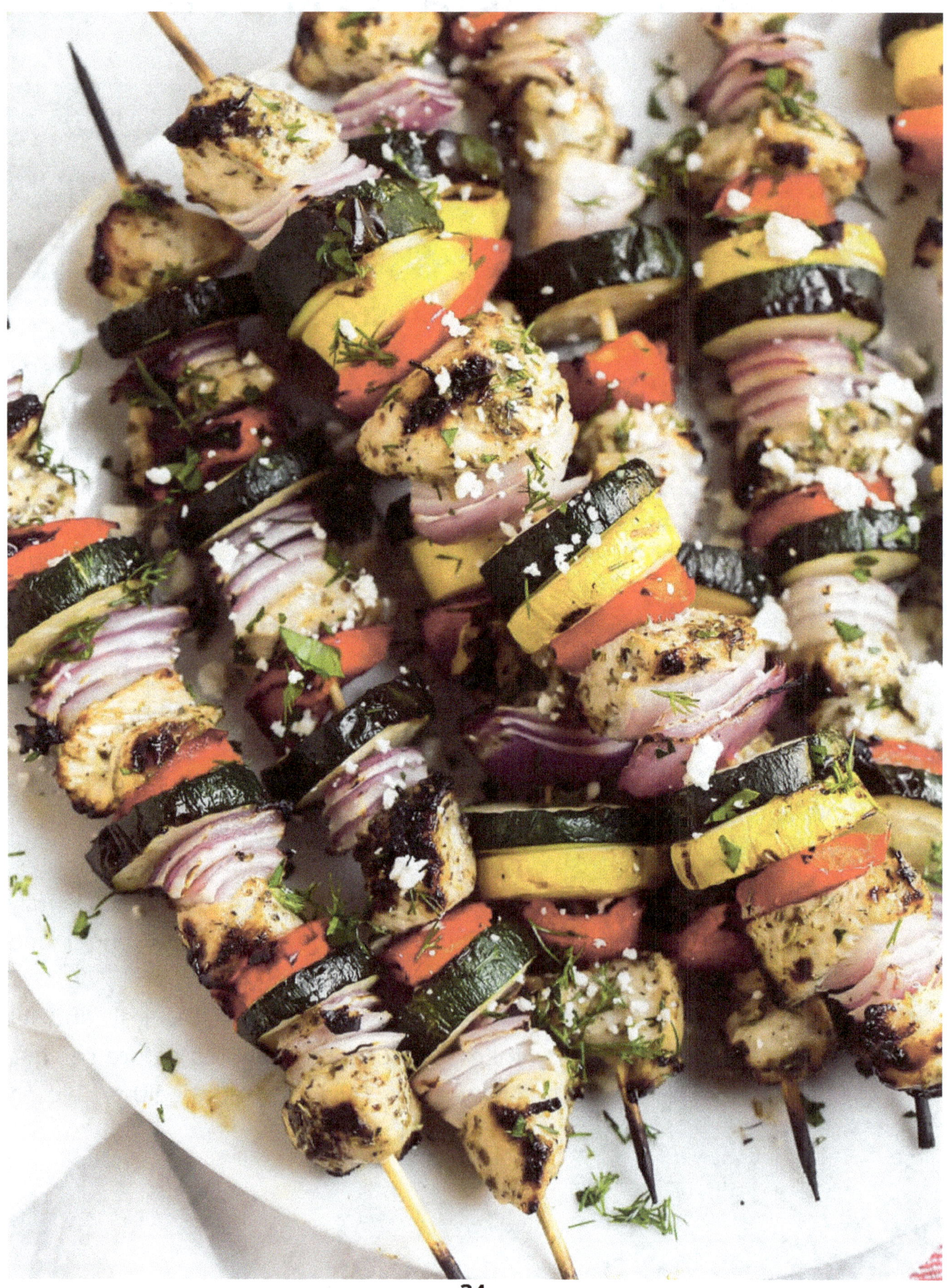

MANGO SALSA

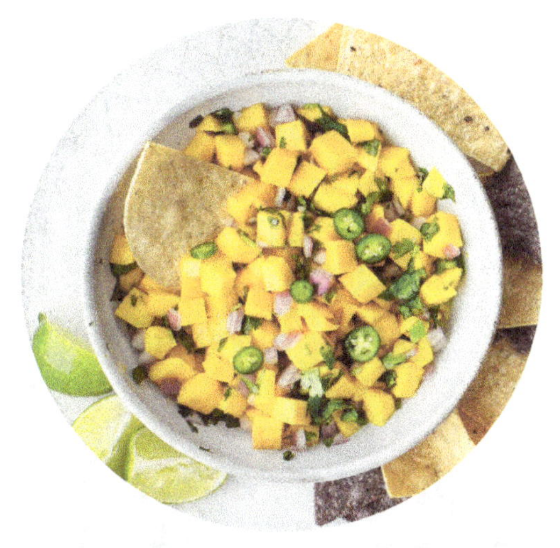

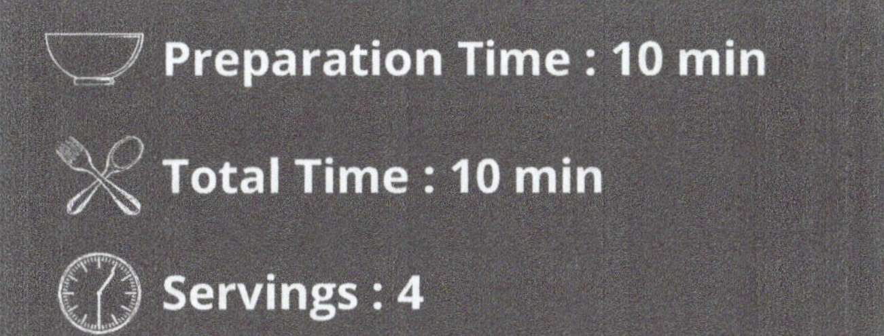

Steps for Cooking

- In a medium bowl, combine the diced mangoes, red bell pepper, red onion, and jalapeño (if using).
- Add the chopped cilantro and lime juice to the bowl. Season with salt to taste.
- Gently toss all the ingredients together until well mixed.
- Serve the mango salsa immediately, or chill in the refrigerator for about 30 minutes to let the flavors meld. Enjoy your fresh and vibrant mango salsa with chips, grilled fish, chicken, or as a topping for tacos!

Ingredients

- 2 ripe mangoes, peeled, pitted, and diced
- 1 red bell pepper, diced
- 1/2 red onion, finely diced
- 1 jalapeño, seeded and finely diced (optional)
- 1/4 cup fresh cilantro, chopped
- 2 tablespoons lime juice
- Salt to taste

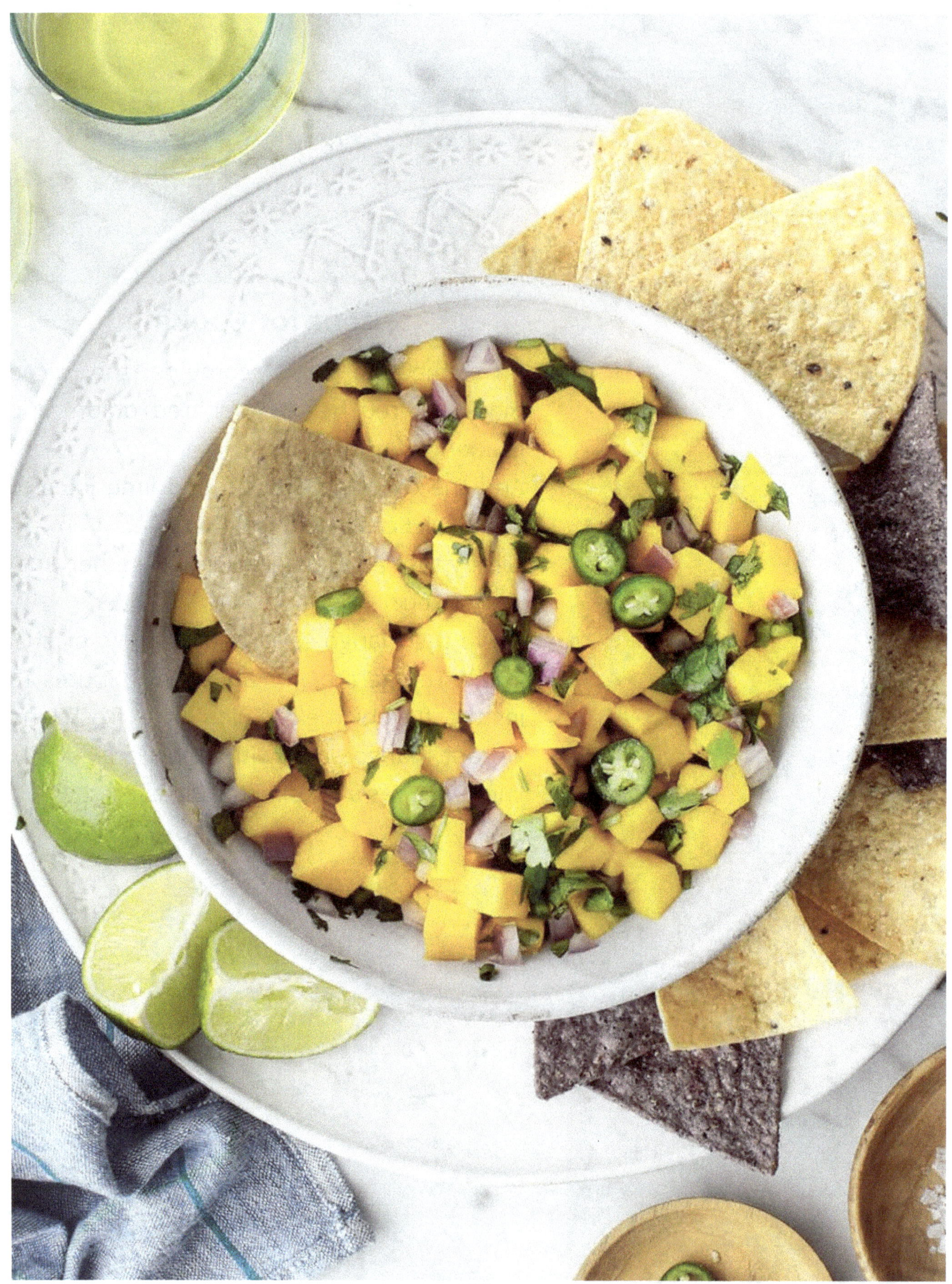

EGGPLANT LASAGNA

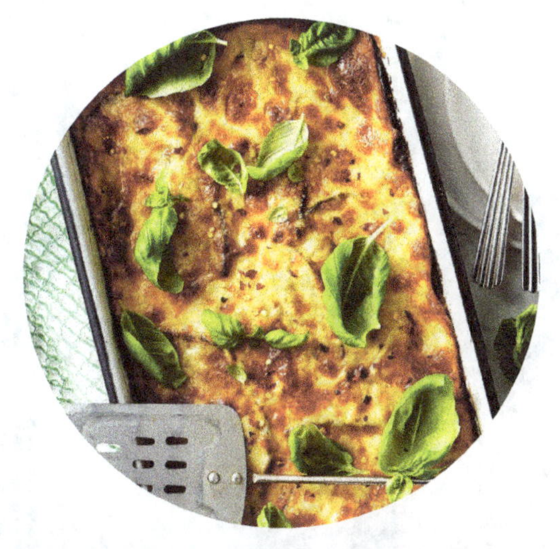

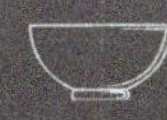 **Preparation Time : 20 min**

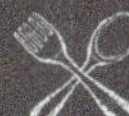 **Total Time : 80 min**

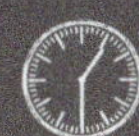 **Servings : 6**

Ingredients

- 2 large eggplants, sliced lengthwise into 1/4-inch thick slices
- 1 tablespoon olive oil
- Salt and pepper to taste
- 1 lb ground turkey or beef
- 1 small onion, diced
- 2 cloves garlic, minced
- 1 jar (24 oz) marinara sauce
- 1 cup ricotta cheese
- 1 large egg
- 2 cups shredded mozzarella cheese
- 1/2 cup grated Parmesan cheese
- Fresh basil or parsley for garnish (optional)

Steps for Cooking

- Preheat oven to 375°F (190°C). Line baking sheets with parchment paper. Brush eggplant slices with olive oil, season with salt and pepper, and roast for 20 minutes, flipping halfway through.
- Cook ground turkey or beef in a skillet over medium heat until browned. Add onion and garlic, cook for 3-4 minutes. Stir in marinara sauce and simmer for 10 minutes.
- Mix ricotta cheese with egg in a bowl.
- Spread a thin layer of meat sauce in a 9x13 inch baking dish. Layer with roasted eggplant slices, ricotta mixture, and mozzarella cheese. Repeat layers, ending with meat sauce and topping with remaining mozzarella and Parmesan cheese.
- Cover with foil and bake for 25 minutes. Remove foil and bake for an additional 10-15 minutes until cheese is bubbly and golden brown.
- Let cool for a few minutes before slicing. Garnish with fresh basil or parsley if desired. Enjoy your eggplant lasagna!

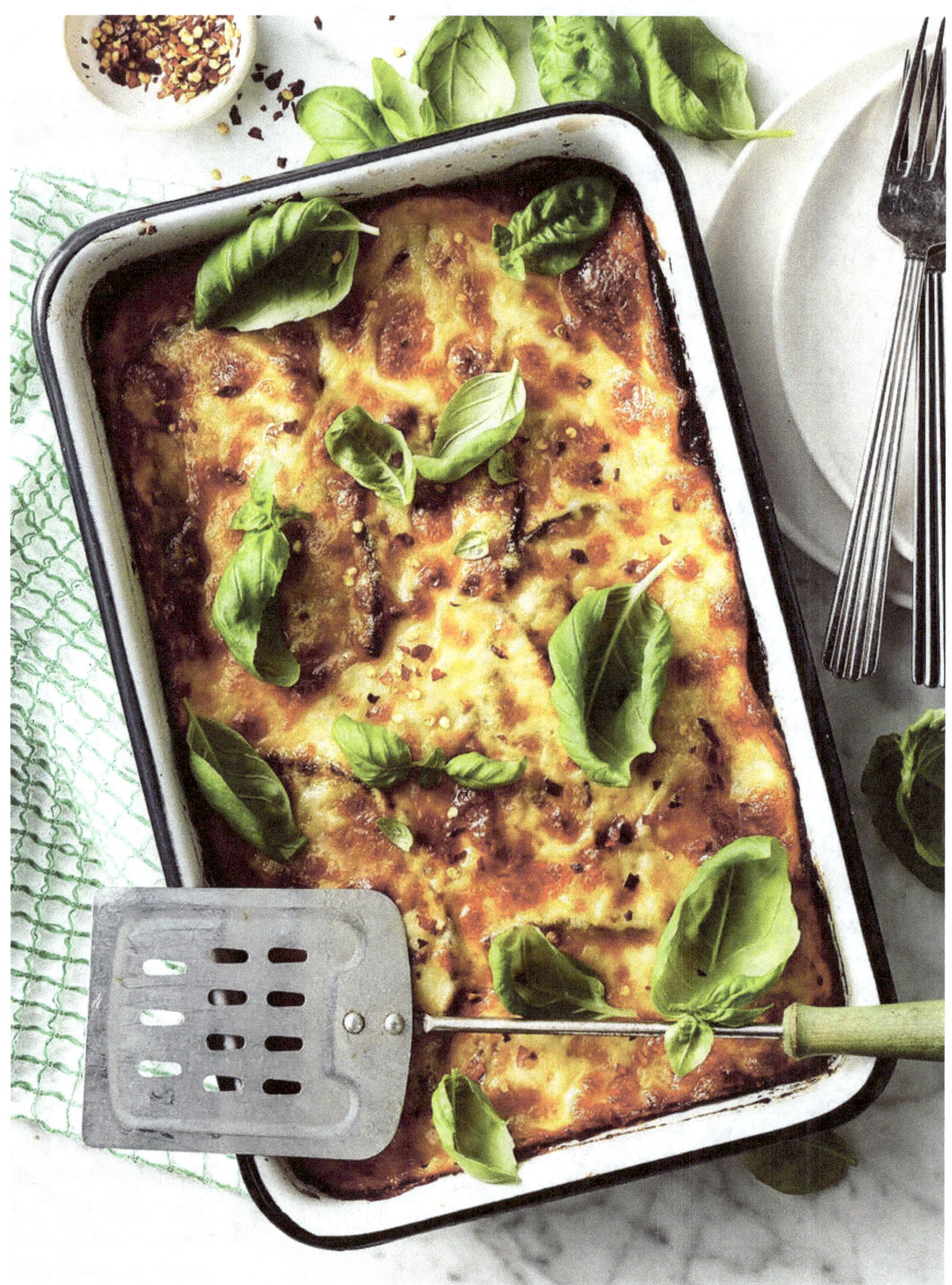

GRILLED PINEAPPLE

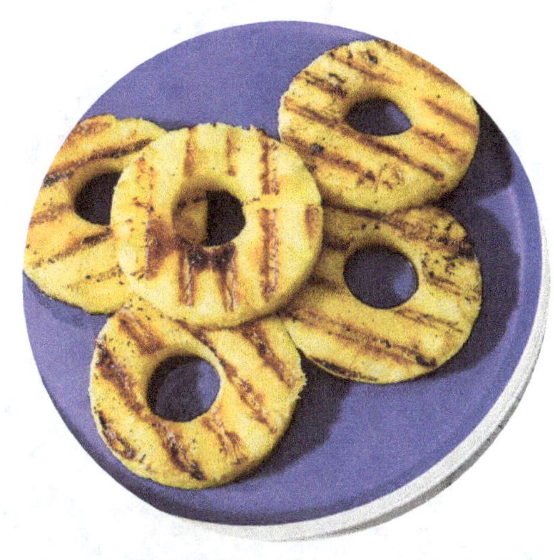

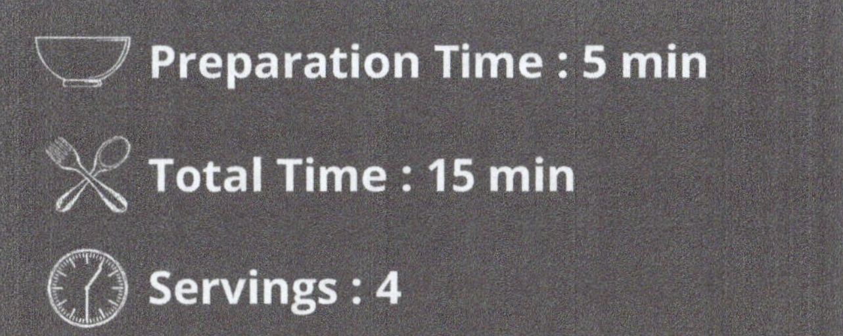

Preparation Time : 5 min

Total Time : 15 min

Servings : 4

Steps for Cooking

- Preheat your grill to medium-high heat.
- If desired, sprinkle the pineapple slices with brown sugar or honey and ground cinnamon for extra sweetness and flavor.
- Place the pineapple slices on the grill and cook for about 3-4 minutes per side, or until grill marks appear and the pineapple is heated through.
- Remove from the grill and serve immediately. Enjoy your delicious and refreshing grilled pineapple!

Ingredients

- 1 fresh pineapple, peeled, cored, and cut into rings or spears
- 2 tablespoons brown sugar or honey (optional)
- 1 teaspoon ground cinnamon (optional)

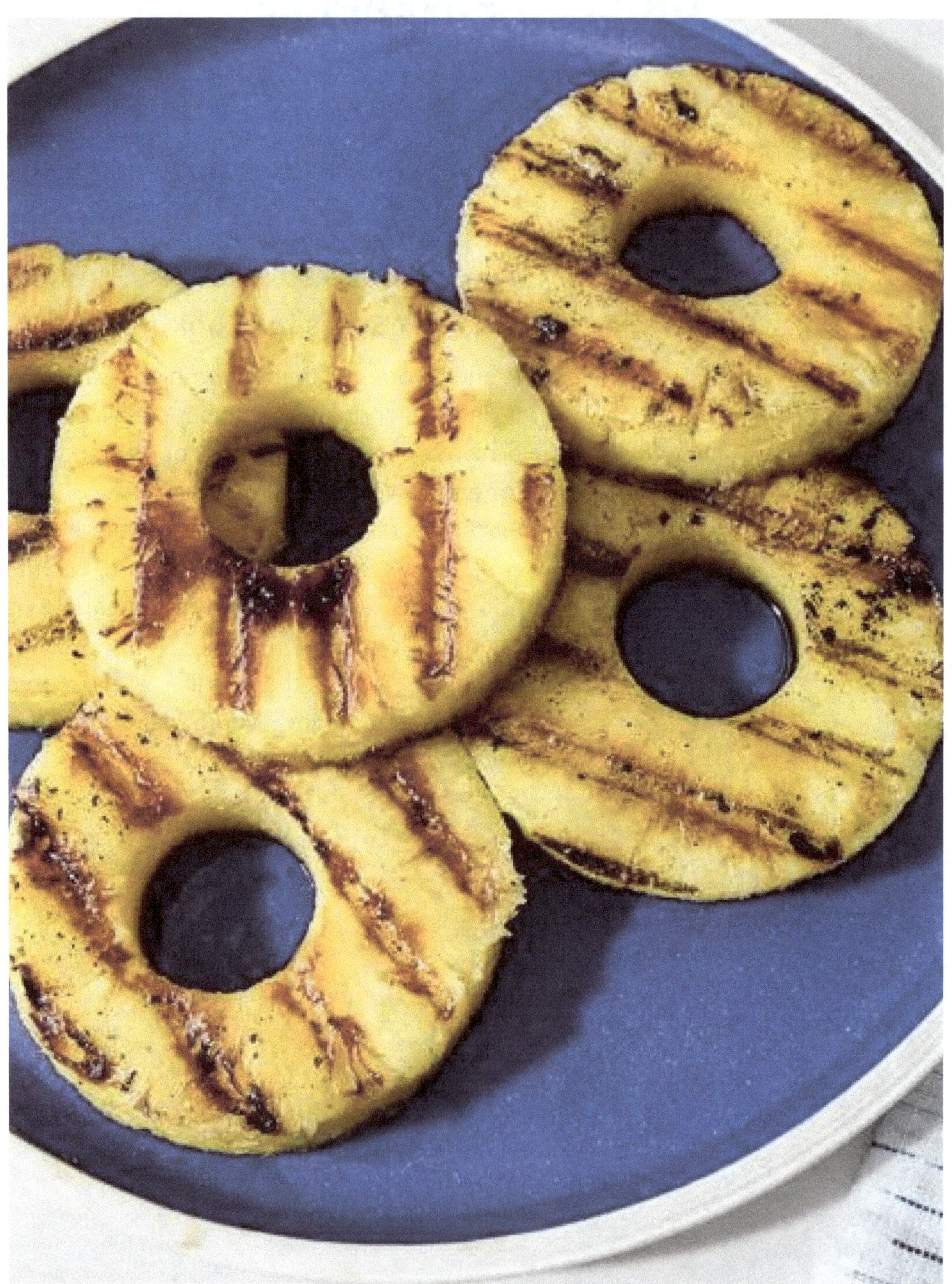

CHICKPEA SALAD

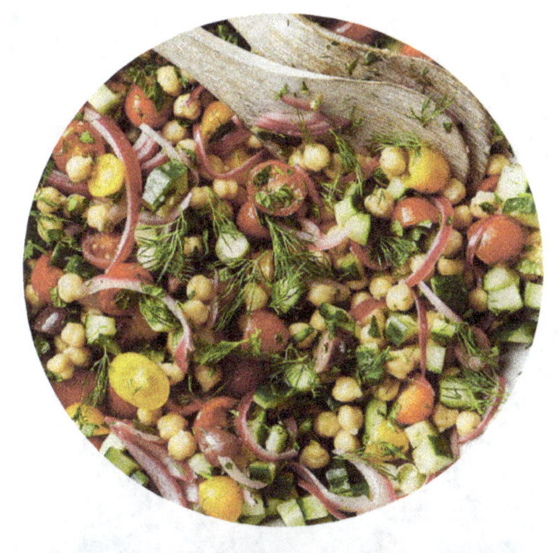

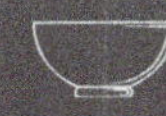 **Preparation Time : 10 min**

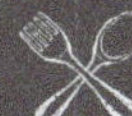 **Total Time : 10 min**

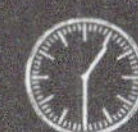 **Servings : 4**

Steps for Cooking

- In a large bowl, combine the chickpeas, cherry tomatoes, cucumber, red onion, and fresh parsley.
- If using, add the crumbled feta cheese to the bowl.
- In a small bowl, whisk together the olive oil, lemon juice, salt, and pepper.
- Pour the dressing over the chickpea mixture and toss to combine thoroughly.
- Serve the chickpea salad immediately, or chill in the refrigerator for about 30 minutes to let the flavors meld. Enjoy your fresh and healthy chickpea salad!

Ingredients

- 1 can (15 oz) chickpeas, drained and rinsed
- 1 cup cherry tomatoes, halved
- 1 cucumber, diced
- 1/4 red onion, finely chopped
- 1/4 cup fresh parsley, chopped
- 1/4 cup feta cheese, crumbled (optional)
- 2 tablespoons olive oil
- 1 tablespoon lemon juice
- Salt and pepper to taste

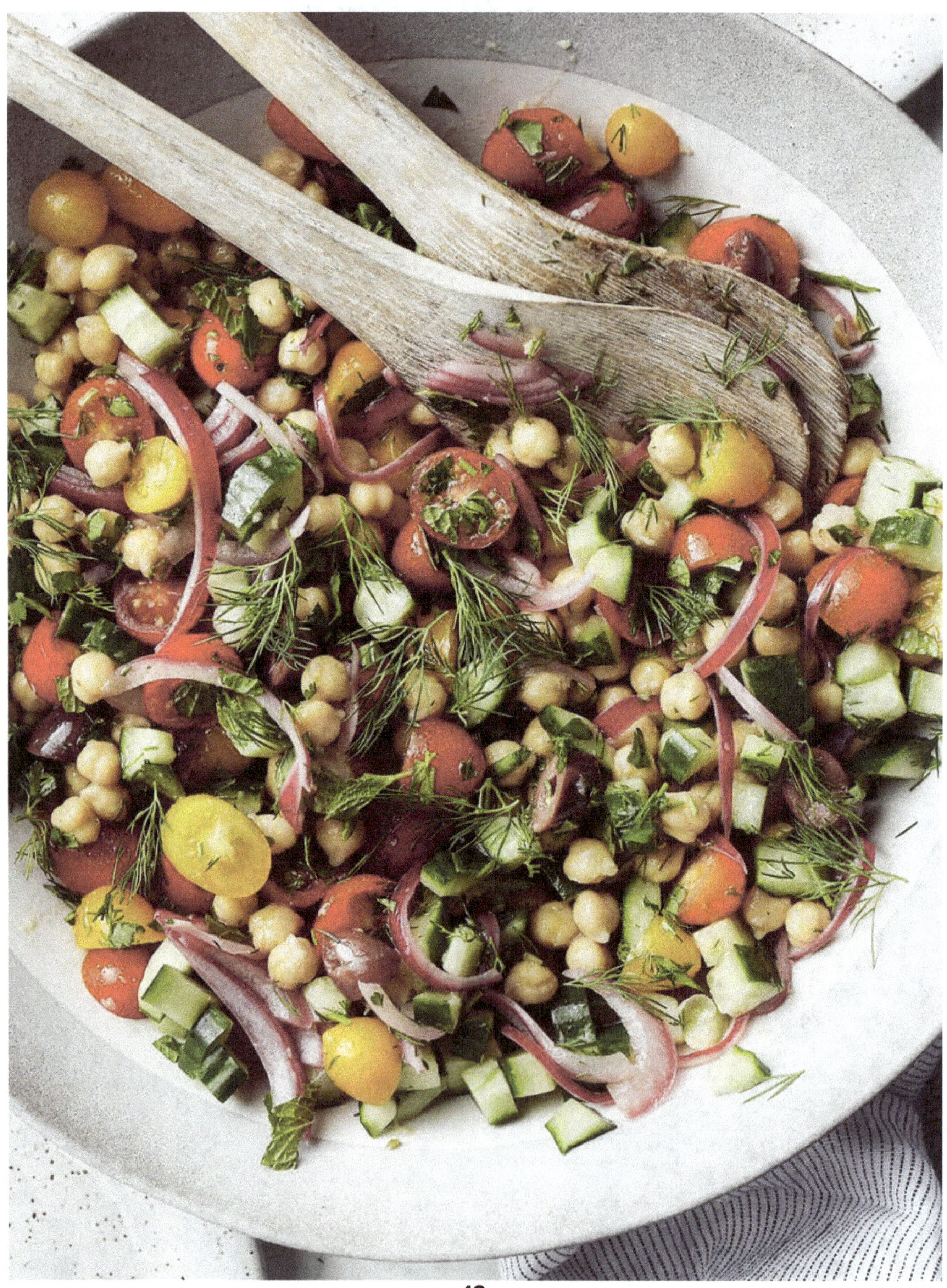

ROASTED CARROT & PARSNIP FRIES

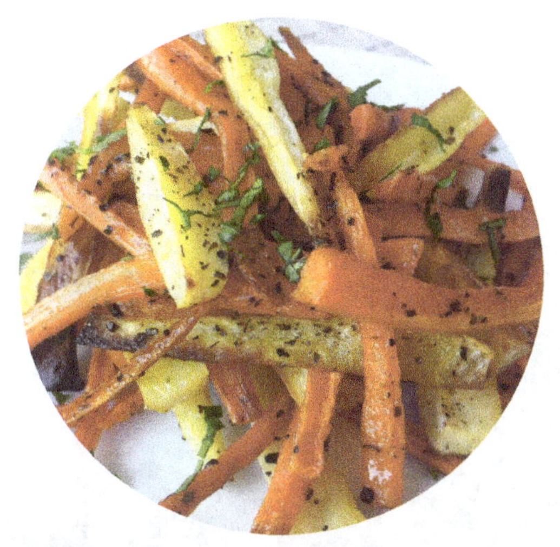

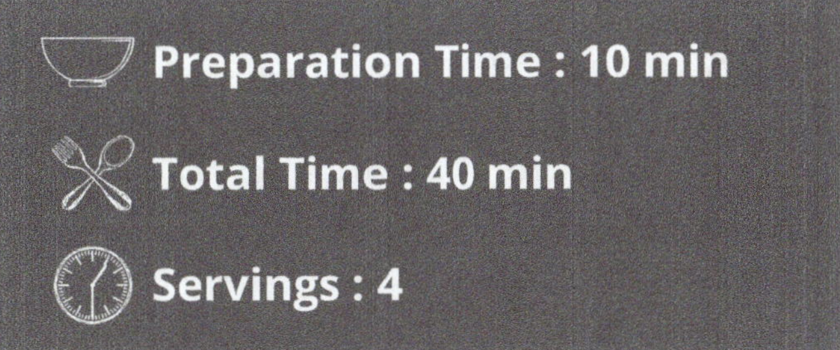

Steps for Cooking

- Preheat your oven to 425°F (220°C). Line a baking sheet with parchment paper.
- In a large bowl, toss the carrot and parsnip fries with olive oil, garlic powder, paprika, salt, and pepper until evenly coated.
- Spread the fries in a single layer on the prepared baking sheet.
- Roast in the preheated oven for 25-30 minutes, turning halfway through, until the fries are tender and lightly browned.
- Remove from the oven and garnish with fresh parsley if desired. Serve immediately and enjoy your healthy and delicious roasted carrot and parsnip fries!

Ingredients

- 4 large carrots, peeled and cut into fries
- 4 large parsnips, peeled and cut into fries
- 2 tablespoons olive oil
- 1 teaspoon garlic powder
- 1 teaspoon paprika
- Salt and pepper to taste
- Fresh parsley, chopped (optional, for garnish)

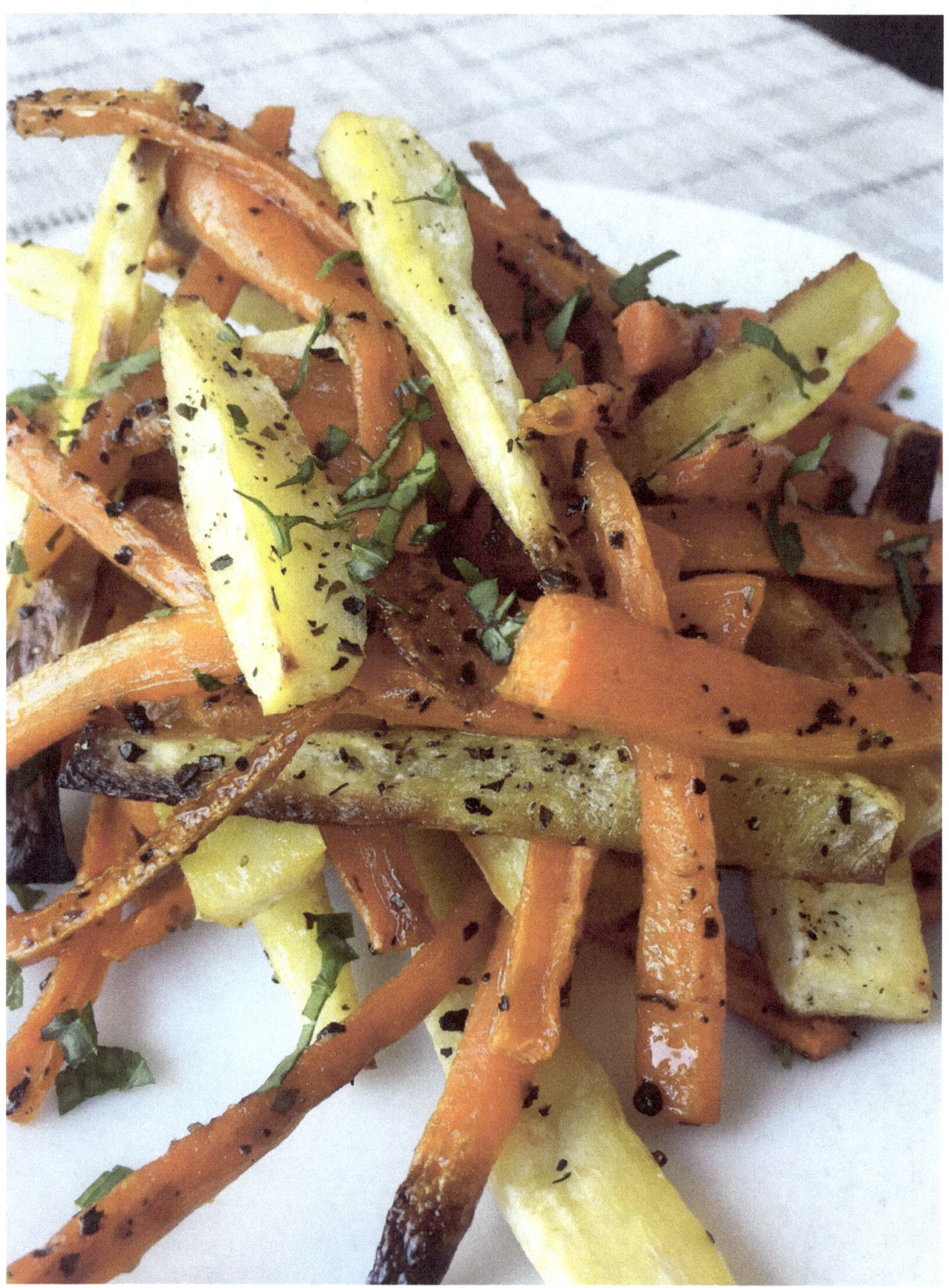

QUINOA & BLACK BEAN SALAD

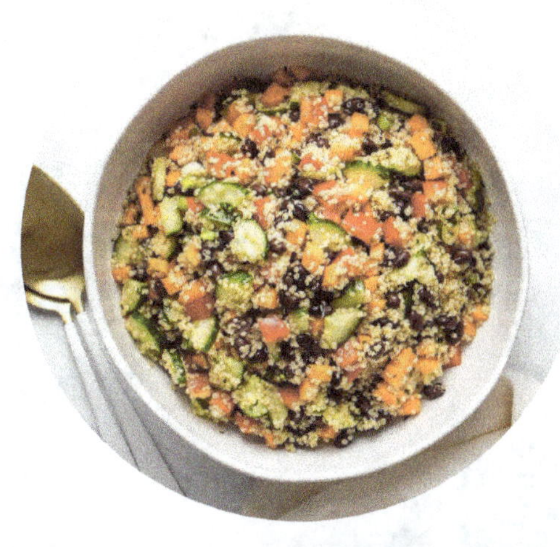

Ingredients

- 1 cup quinoa
- 2 cups water
- 1 can (15 oz) black beans, drained and rinsed
- 1 cup corn kernels (fresh, frozen, or canned)
- 1 red bell pepper, diced
- 1/4 red onion, finely chopped
- 1/4 cup fresh cilantro, chopped
- 1/4 cup olive oil
- 2 tablespoons lime juice
- 1 teaspoon ground cumin
- Salt and pepper to taste

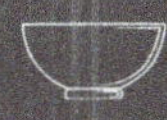 **Preparation Time : 10 min**

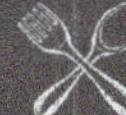 **Total Time : 30 min**

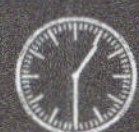 **Servings : 4**

Steps for Cooking

- Start by rinsing the quinoa under cold water. In a medium saucepan, bring the quinoa and water to a boil. Reduce the heat to low, cover, and simmer for about 15 minutes or until the water is absorbed and the quinoa is tender. Remove from heat and let it cool.
- In a large bowl, combine the cooked quinoa, black beans, corn, diced red bell pepper, and finely chopped red onion.
- In a small bowl, whisk together the olive oil, lime juice, ground cumin, salt, and pepper.
- Pour the dressing over the quinoa mixture and toss to combine thoroughly.
- Garnish with fresh cilantro and serve the quinoa and black bean salad immediately, or chill in the refrigerator for about 30 minutes to let the flavors meld. Enjoy your nutritious and delicious quinoa and black bean salad!

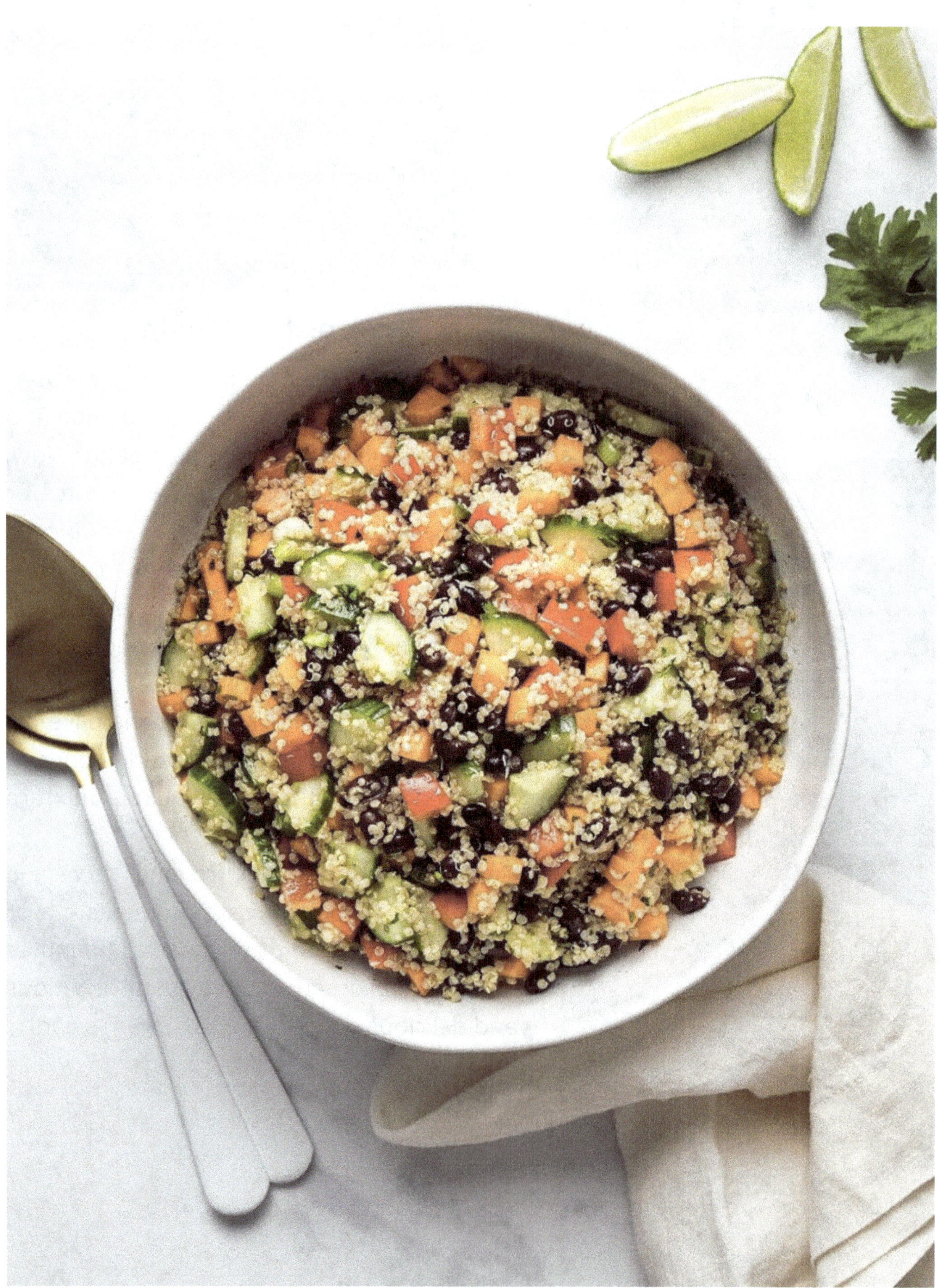

STUFFED MUSHROOMS

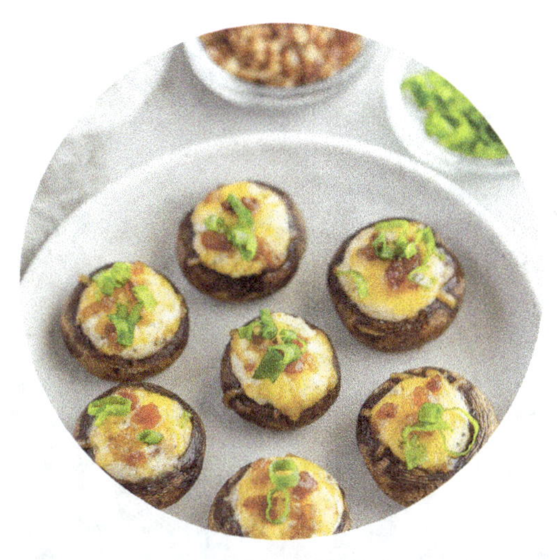

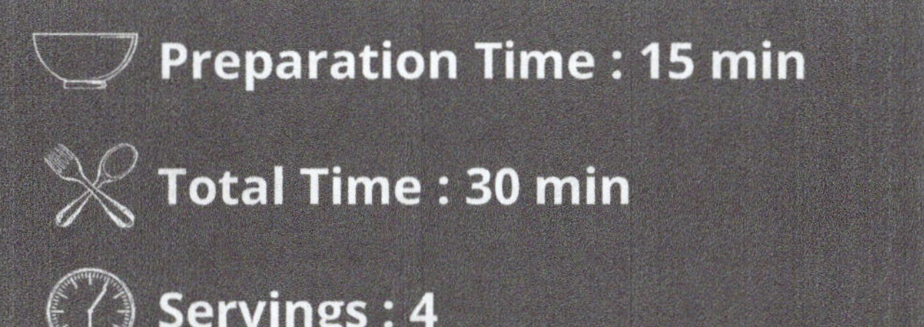

Ingredients

- 16 large white or cremini mushrooms
- 2 tablespoons olive oil
- 1 small onion, finely chopped
- 2 cloves garlic, minced
- 1/4 cup breadcrumbs
- 1/4 cup grated Parmesan cheese
- 1/4 cup cream cheese, softened
- 2 tablespoons fresh parsley, chopped
- Salt and pepper to taste

Steps for Cooking

- Preheat your oven to 375°F (190°C). Line a baking sheet with parchment paper.
- Clean the mushrooms and remove the stems, finely chopping the stems and setting them aside.
- In a skillet, heat the olive oil over medium heat. Add the chopped mushroom stems, onion, and garlic, cooking for about 5 minutes until softened.
- In a bowl, combine the cooked mushroom mixture with breadcrumbs, Parmesan cheese, cream cheese, chopped parsley, salt, and pepper. Mix until well combined.
- Stuff each mushroom cap with the filling mixture and place them on the prepared baking sheet.
- Bake in the preheated oven for 15-20 minutes, or until the mushrooms are tender and the filling is golden brown.
- Serve the stuffed mushrooms hot, and enjoy your delicious appetizer!

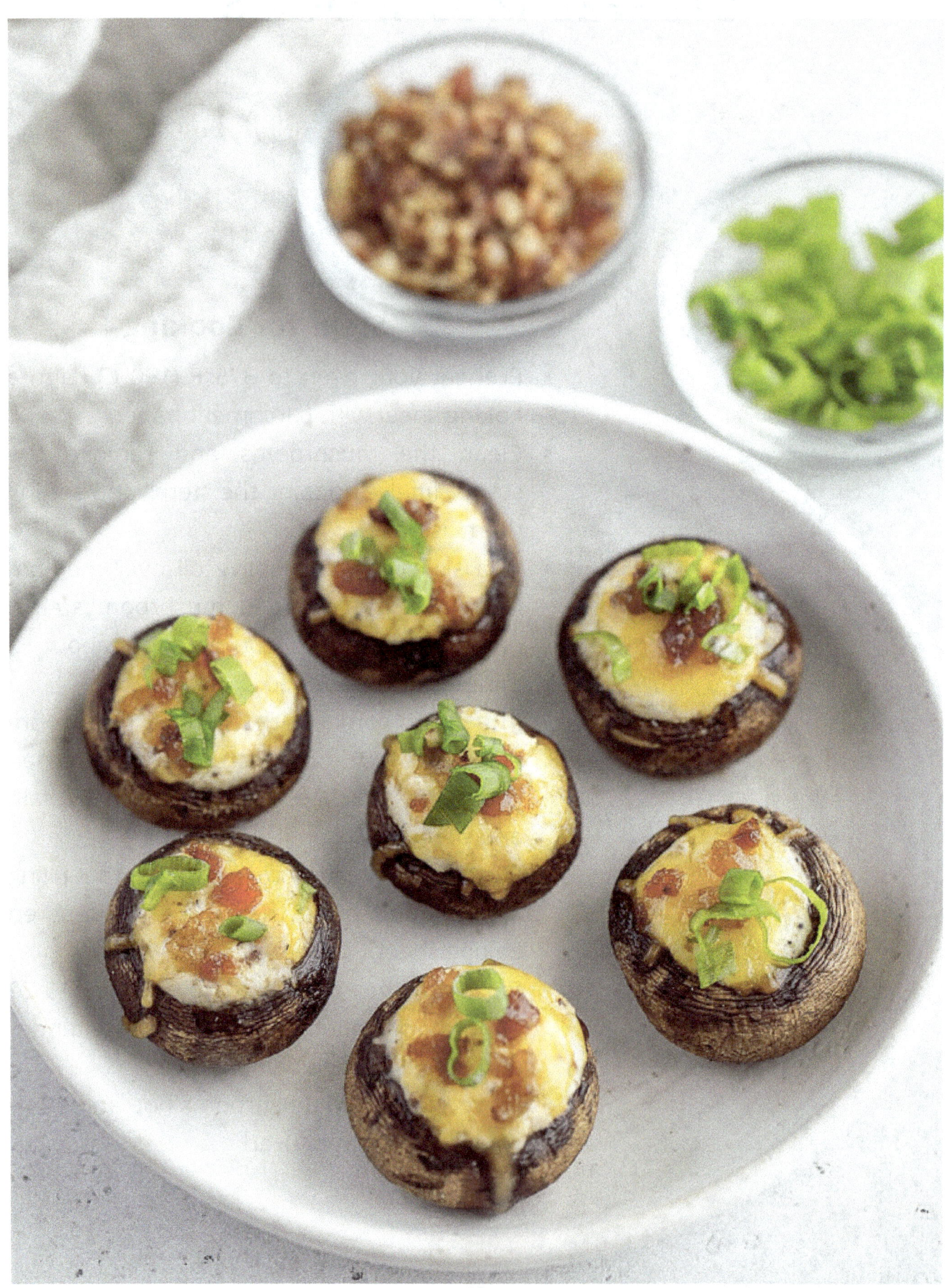

LENTIL SOUP

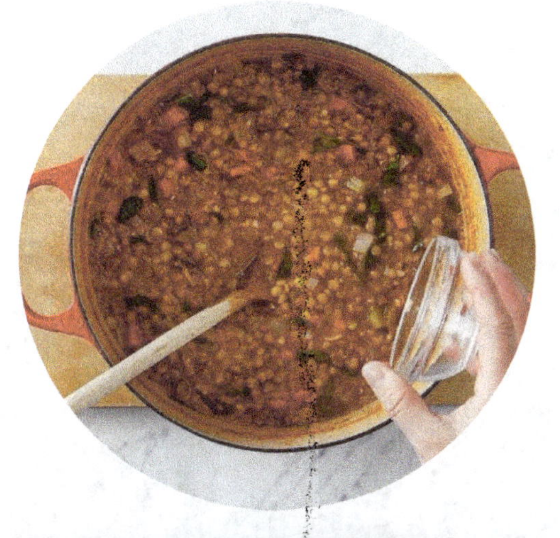

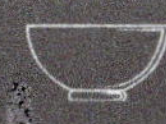
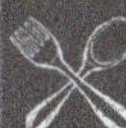
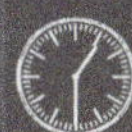

Ingredients

- 1 tablespoon olive oil
- 1 onion, diced
- 2 carrots, diced
- 2 celery stalks, diced
- 3 cloves garlic, minced
- 1 teaspoon ground cumin
- 1 teaspoon ground coriander
- 1 teaspoon smoked paprika
- 1 cup dried lentils, rinsed and drained
- 1 can (14.5 oz) diced tomatoes
- 6 cups vegetable broth
- 2 bay leaves
- Salt and pepper to taste
- 2 cups fresh spinach or kale, chopped (optional)
- Fresh lemon juice, for serving (optional)

Steps for Cooking

- Start by heating the olive oil in a large pot over medium heat. Add the diced onion, carrots, and celery, and cook for about 5 minutes until softened.
- Stir in the minced garlic, ground cumin, ground coriander, and smoked paprika, cooking for another 1-2 minutes until fragrant.
- Add the rinsed lentils, diced tomatoes, vegetable broth, and bay leaves to the pot. Bring to a boil, then reduce the heat and let it simmer for about 25-30 minutes until the lentils are tender.
- Season with salt and pepper to taste. If using, stir in the chopped spinach or kale and cook for an additional 2-3 minutes until wilted.
- Remove the bay leaves and stir in a squeeze of fresh lemon juice if desired.
- Serve the lentil soup hot, garnished with chopped fresh parsley if desired. Enjoy your hearty and nutritious lentil soup!

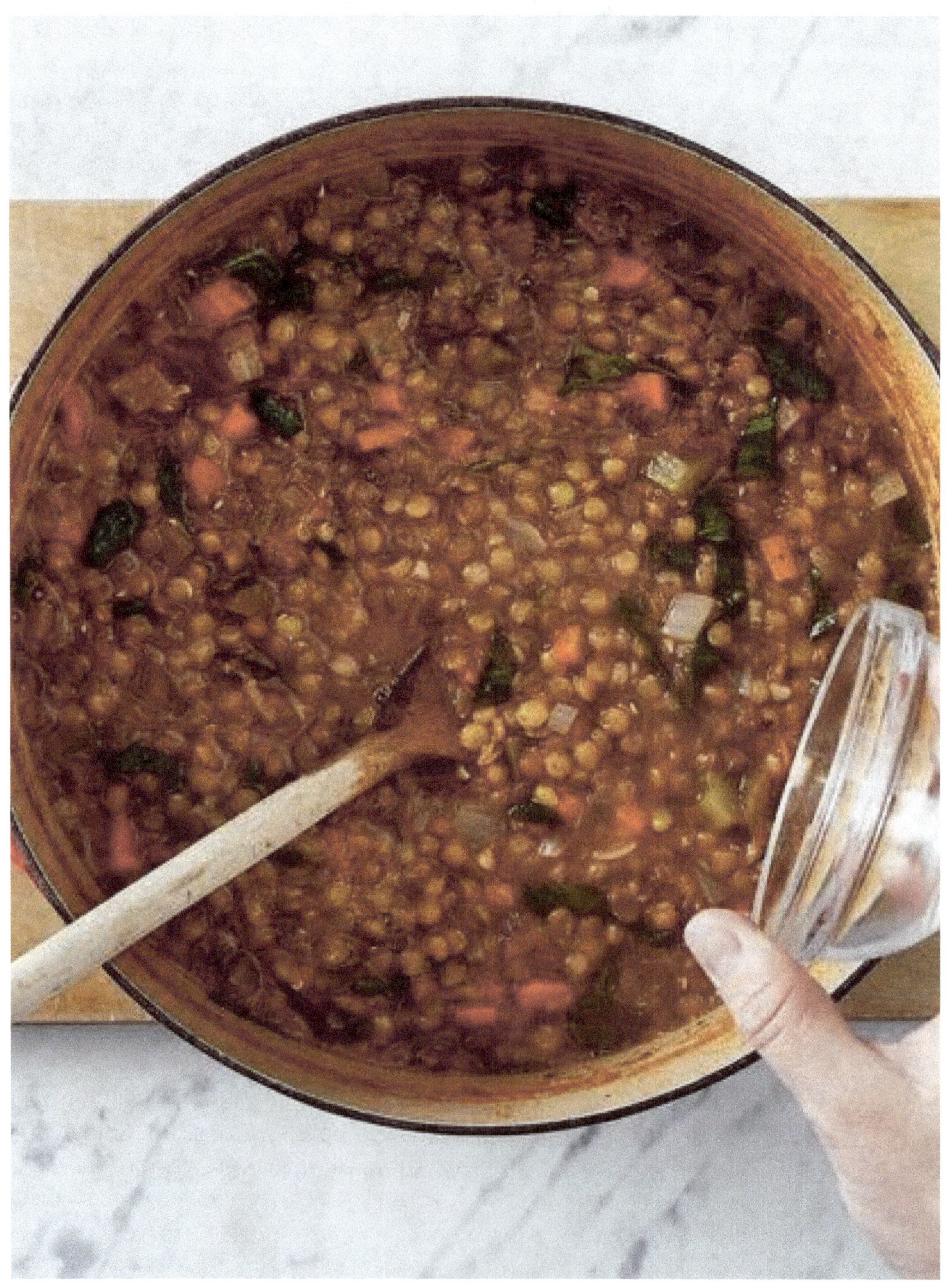

BERRY SMOOTHIE

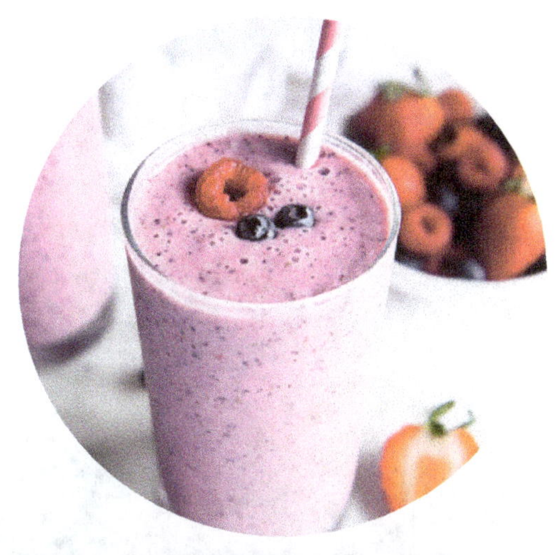

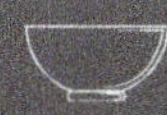 **Preparation Time : 5 min**

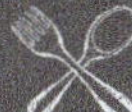 **Total Time : 5 min**

 **Servings : 2**

Ingredients

- 1 cup mixed berries (fresh or frozen)
- 1 banana
- 1/2 cup Greek yogurt
- 1/2 cup milk (or any plant-based milk)
- 1 tablespoon honey (optional)
- 1/2 teaspoon vanilla extract (optional)
- Ice cubes (optional, for a thicker smoothie)

Steps for Cooking

- In a blender, combine the mixed berries, banana, Greek yogurt, milk, honey, and vanilla extract.
- Blend until smooth. If you prefer a thicker consistency, add a few ice cubes and blend again.
- Pour the smoothie into glasses and serve immediately. Enjoy your refreshing and healthy berry smoothie!

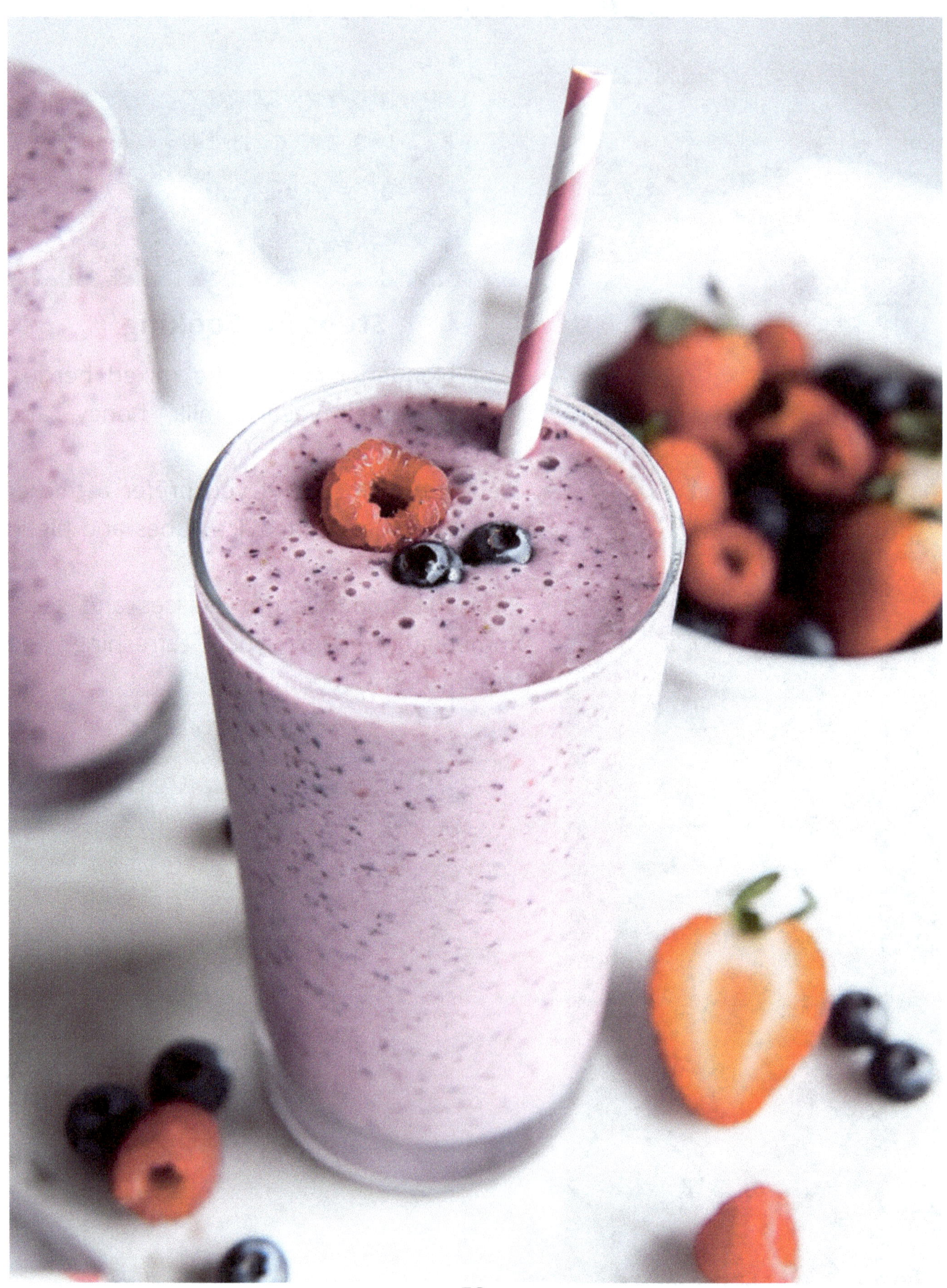

CUCUMBER & TOMATO SALAD

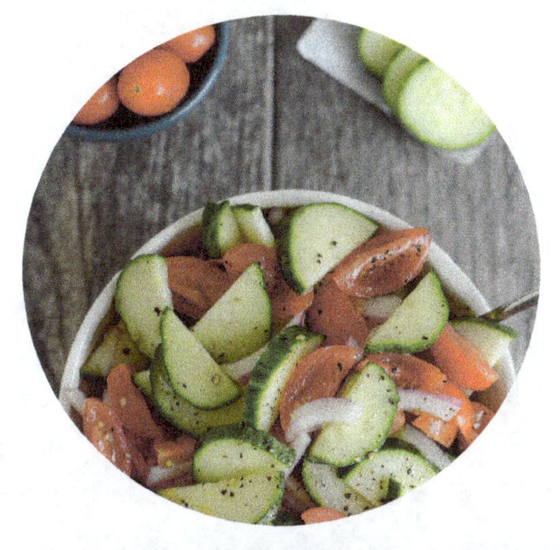

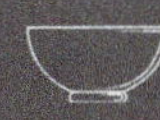 **Preparation Time : 10 min**

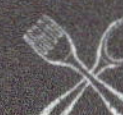 **Total Time : 10 min**

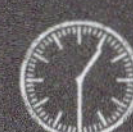 **Servings : 4**

Ingredients

- 2 cucumbers, sliced
- 4 tomatoes, diced
- 1/4 red onion, thinly sliced
- 1/4 cup fresh parsley, chopped
- 2 tablespoons olive oil
- 1 tablespoon red wine vinegar
- Salt and pepper to taste

Steps for Cooking

- In a large bowl, combine the sliced cucumbers, diced tomatoes, thinly sliced red onion, and chopped fresh parsley.
- In a small bowl, whisk together the olive oil, red wine vinegar, salt, and pepper.
- Pour the dressing over the cucumber and tomato mixture. Toss gently to combine and ensure everything is evenly coated.
- Serve the cucumber and tomato salad immediately, or chill in the refrigerator for about 30 minutes to let the flavors meld. Enjoy your fresh and healthy salad!

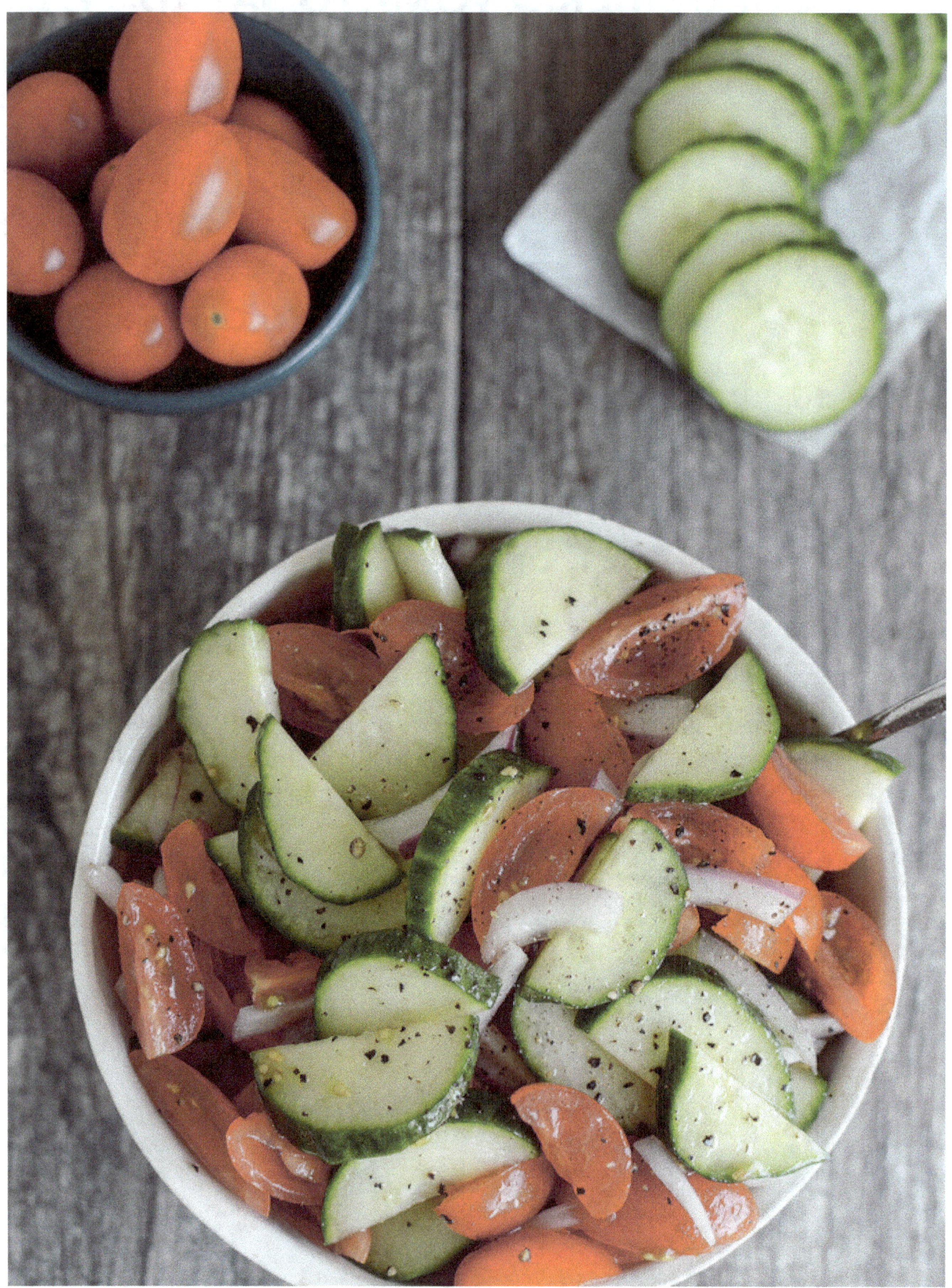

ROASTED BRUSSELS SPROUTS

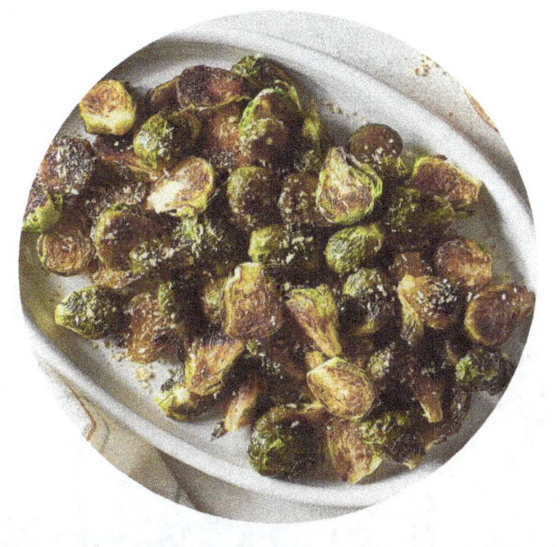

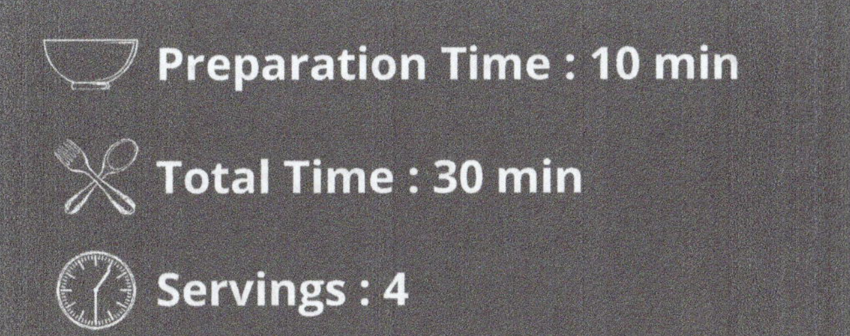

Ingredients

- 1 lb Brussels sprouts, trimmed and halved
- 2 tablespoons olive oil
- Salt and pepper to taste
- Optional: 1 tablespoon balsamic vinegar or lemon juice for extra flavor

Steps for Cooking

- Preheat your oven to 400°F (200°C). Line a baking sheet with parchment paper.
- In a large bowl, toss the halved Brussels sprouts with olive oil, salt, and pepper until evenly coated.
- Spread the Brussels sprouts in a single layer on the prepared baking sheet.
- Roast in the preheated oven for 20-25 minutes, turning halfway through, until the Brussels sprouts are tender and caramelized.
- If desired, drizzle with balsamic vinegar or lemon juice before serving.
- Serve the roasted Brussels sprouts hot, and enjoy your delicious and healthy side dish!

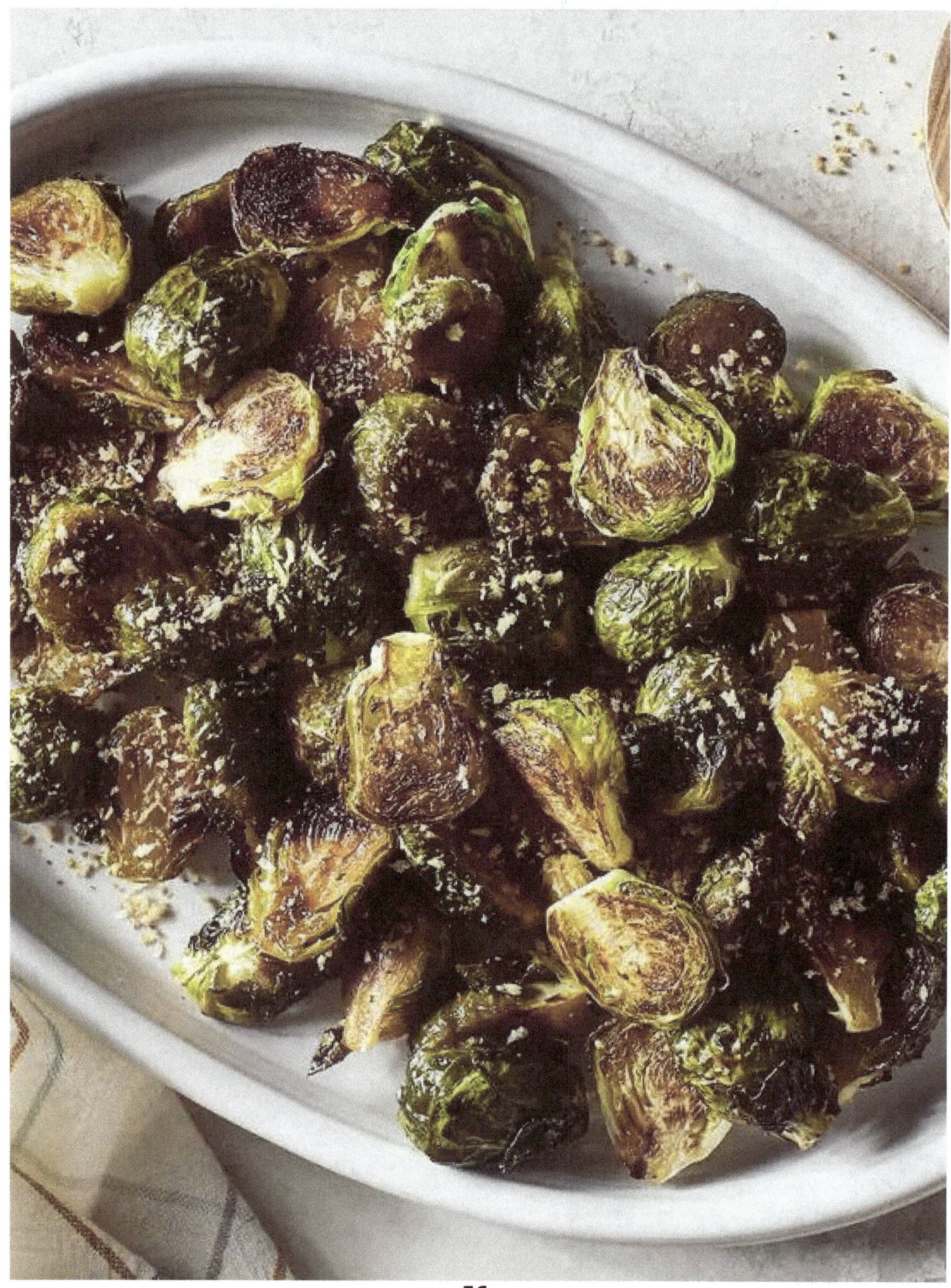

CHICKEN & CABBAGE STIR-FRY

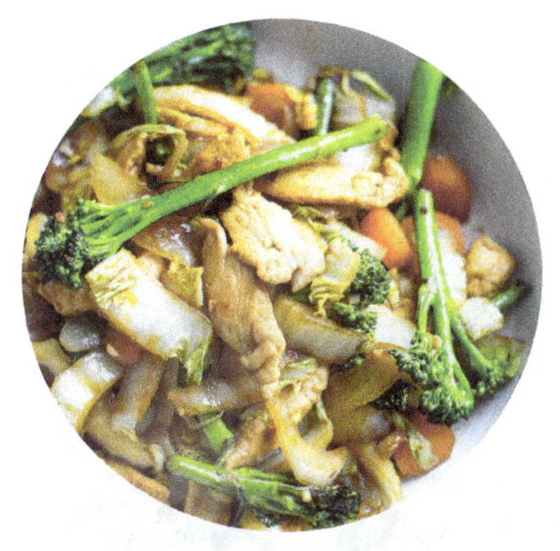

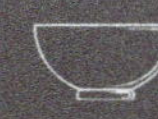
Preparation Time : 15 min

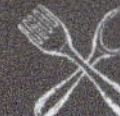
Total Time : 30 min

Servings : 4

Steps for Cooking

- In a large skillet or wok, heat the vegetable oil over medium-high heat. Add the thinly sliced chicken breasts and cook until no longer pink, about 5-7 minutes. Remove the chicken from the skillet and set it aside.
- In the same skillet, add the sesame oil. Sauté the minced garlic and ginger for about 1 minute until fragrant.
- Add the thinly sliced cabbage, julienned carrot, and bell pepper to the skillet. Stir-fry for 5-7 minutes until the vegetables are tender but still crisp.
- Return the cooked chicken to the skillet and pour in the soy sauce. Toss everything together and cook for another 2-3 minutes until heated through.
- Season with salt and pepper to taste. Garnish with sliced green onions and sesame seeds if desired.
- Serve the chicken and cabbage stir-fry hot, and enjoy your healthy and flavorful meal!

Ingredients

- 1 lb boneless, skinless chicken breasts, thinly sliced
- 1 small head of cabbage, thinly sliced
- 1 carrot, julienned
- 1 bell pepper, thinly sliced
- 2 cloves garlic, minced
- 2 tablespoons soy sauce
- 1 tablespoon sesame oil
- 1 tablespoon vegetable oil
- 1 tablespoon ginger, minced
- Salt and pepper to taste
- Green onions, sliced (optional, for garnish)
- Sesame seeds (optional, for garnish)

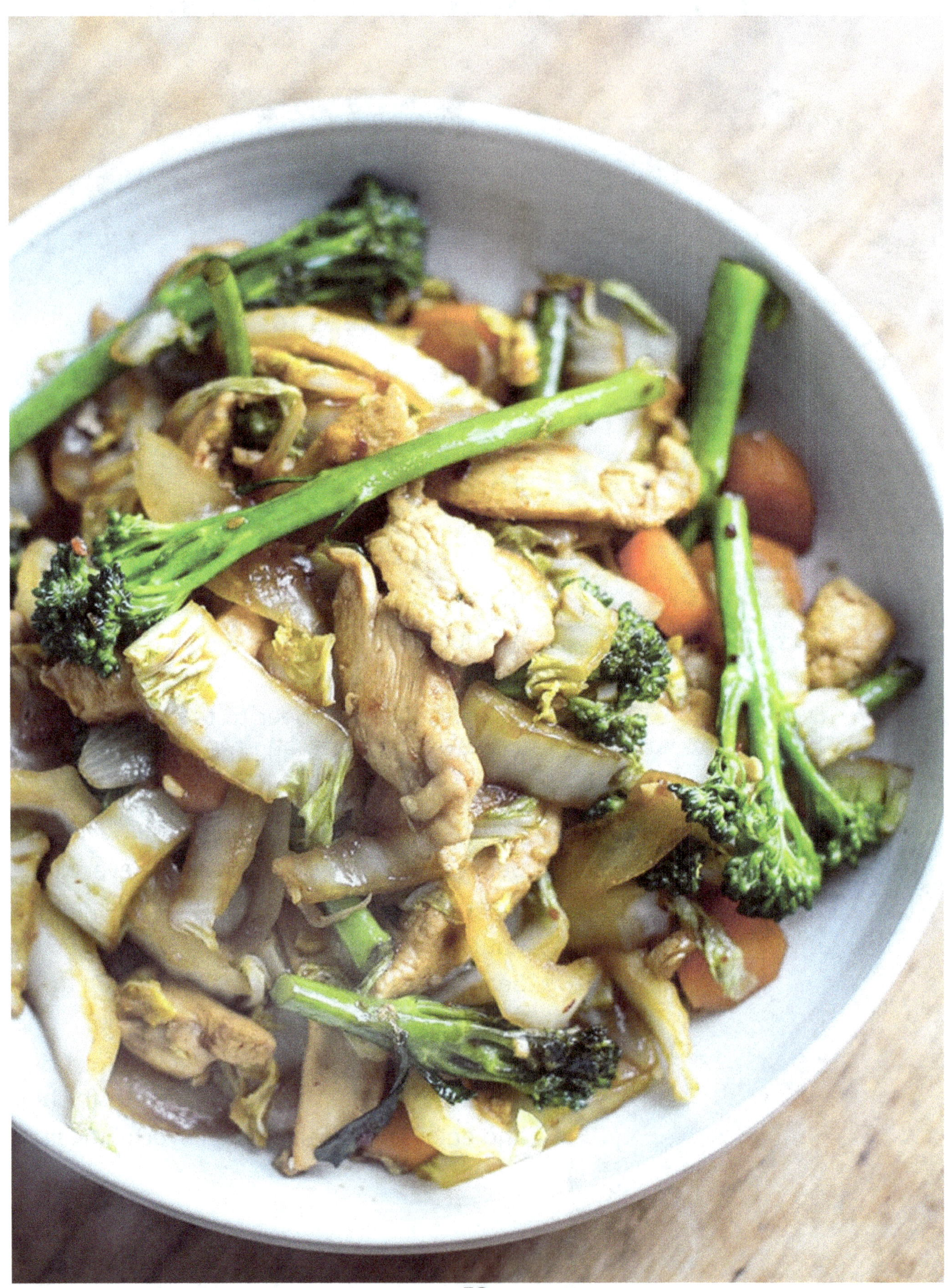

GRILLED VEGGIE SKEWERS

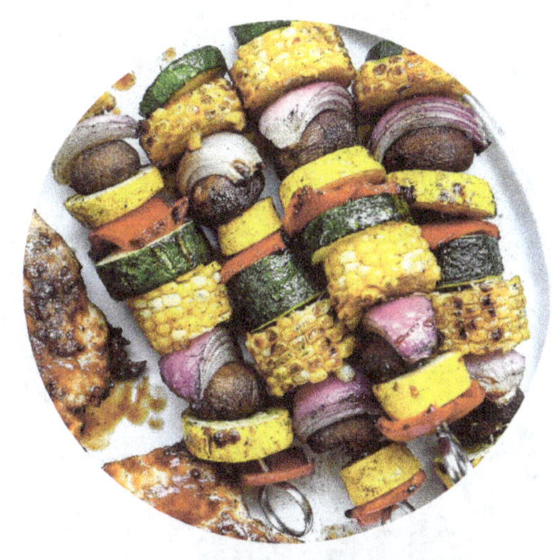

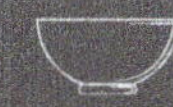**Preparation Time : 15 min**

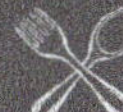**Total Time : 30 min**

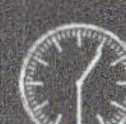**Servings : 4**

Ingredients

- 1 red bell pepper, cut into 1-inch pieces
- 1 yellow bell pepper, cut into 1-inch pieces
- 1 zucchini, sliced into 1/2-inch rounds
- 1 red onion, cut into wedges
- 8 oz mushrooms, halved
- 1/4 cup olive oil
- 2 tablespoons balsamic vinegar
- 2 cloves garlic, minced
- 1 teaspoon dried oregano
- Salt and pepper to taste
- Wooden or metal skewers

Steps for Cooking

- If using wooden skewers, soak them in water for at least 30 minutes to prevent burning.
- In a large bowl, whisk together the olive oil, balsamic vinegar, minced garlic, dried oregano, salt, and pepper.
- Add the bell peppers, zucchini, red onion, and mushrooms to the bowl, tossing to coat them evenly with the marinade. Let it sit for about 10 minutes to absorb the flavors.
- Preheat your grill to medium-high heat.
- Thread the marinated vegetables onto the skewers, alternating between different types of veggies for a colorful mix.
- Place the skewers on the grill and cook for about 10-12 minutes, turning occasionally, until the vegetables are tender and slightly charred.
- Remove from the grill and serve immediately. Enjoy your delicious and healthy grilled veggie skewers!

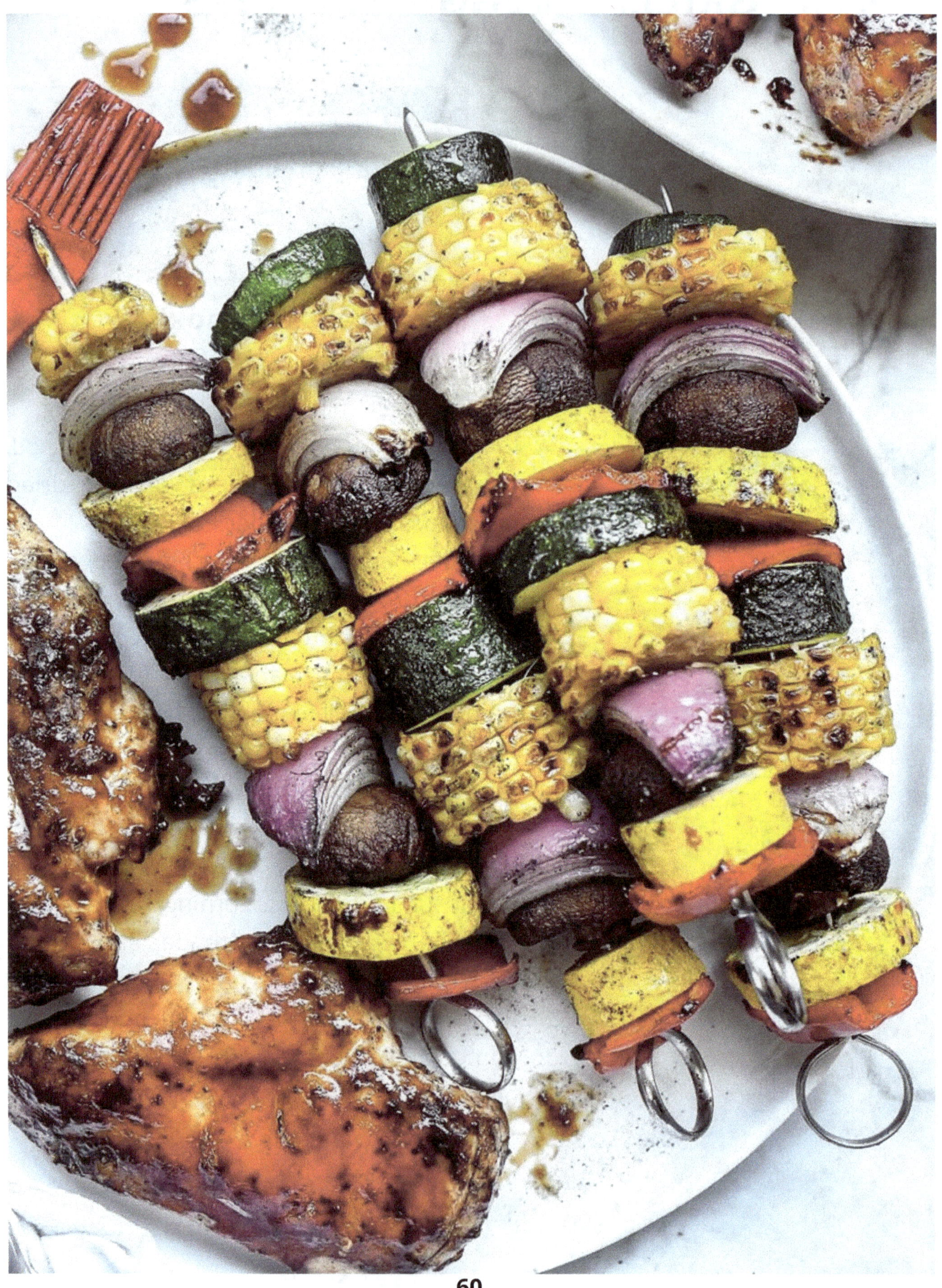

SPINACH & STRAWBERRY SALAD

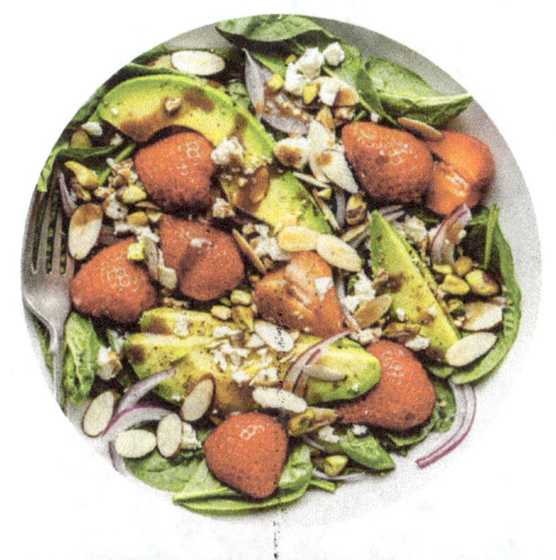

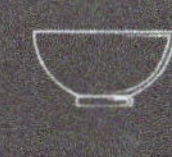 **Preparation Time : 10 min**

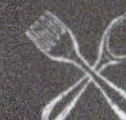 **Total Time : 10 min**

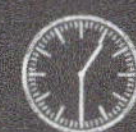 **Servings : 4**

Ingredients

- 6 cups fresh spinach leaves
- 1 cup strawberries, hulled and sliced
- 1/4 red onion, thinly sliced
- 1/4 cup feta cheese, crumbled (optional)
- 1/4 cup sliced almonds or walnuts, toasted (optional)
- 2 tablespoons balsamic vinegar
- 2 tablespoons olive oil
- 1 tablespoon honey (optional)
- Salt and pepper to taste

Steps for Cooking

- In a large bowl, combine the fresh spinach leaves, sliced strawberries, and thinly sliced red onion. If using, add the crumbled feta cheese and toasted nuts.
- In a small bowl, whisk together the balsamic vinegar, olive oil, honey (if using), salt, and pepper.
- Pour the dressing over the salad and toss gently to combine, ensuring all ingredients are evenly coated.
- Serve the spinach and strawberry salad immediately, and enjoy your fresh and flavorful dish!

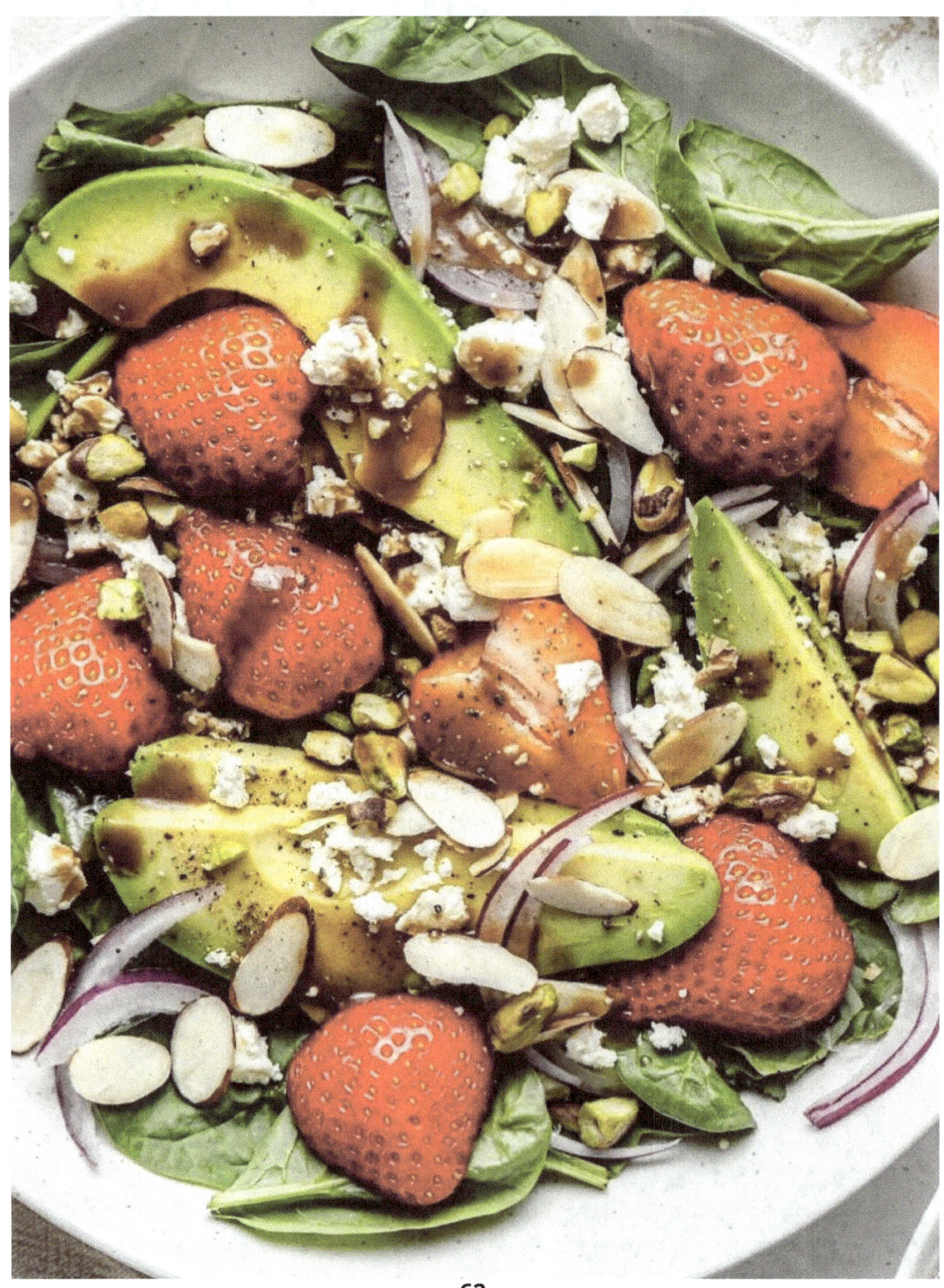

OVEN-BAKED APPLE CHIPS

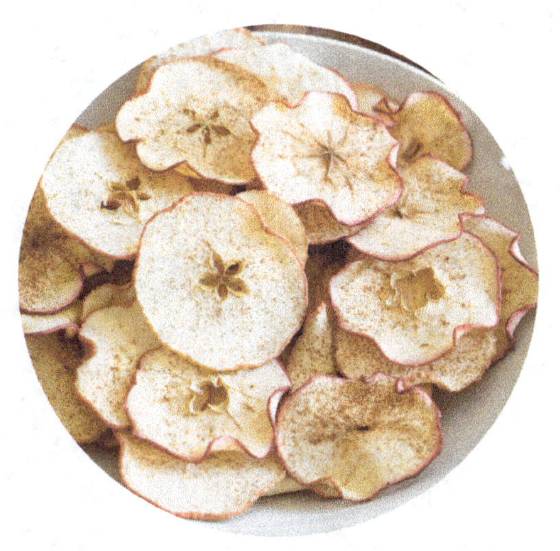

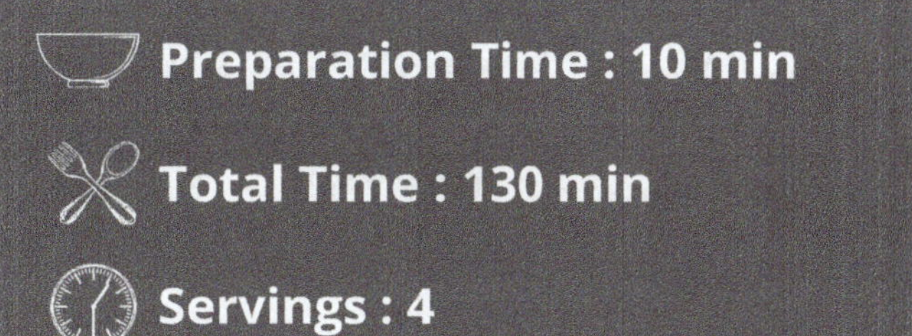

Ingredients

- 2 large apples (any variety)
- 1 teaspoon ground cinnamon (optional)
- 1 tablespoon sugar (optional)

Steps for Cooking

- Preheat your oven to 200°F (95°C). Line two baking sheets with parchment paper.
- Core the apples and slice them thinly using a mandoline or a sharp knife to ensure even slices.
- Arrange the apple slices in a single layer on the prepared baking sheets. If desired, mix the ground cinnamon and sugar in a small bowl and sprinkle over the apple slices.
- Bake in the preheated oven for about 2 hours, turning the slices halfway through, until the apples are dried and crisp. Check occasionally to avoid burning.
- Remove from the oven and let the apple chips cool completely on the baking sheets. They will continue to crisp up as they cool.
- Enjoy your healthy and delicious oven-baked apple chips as a snack!

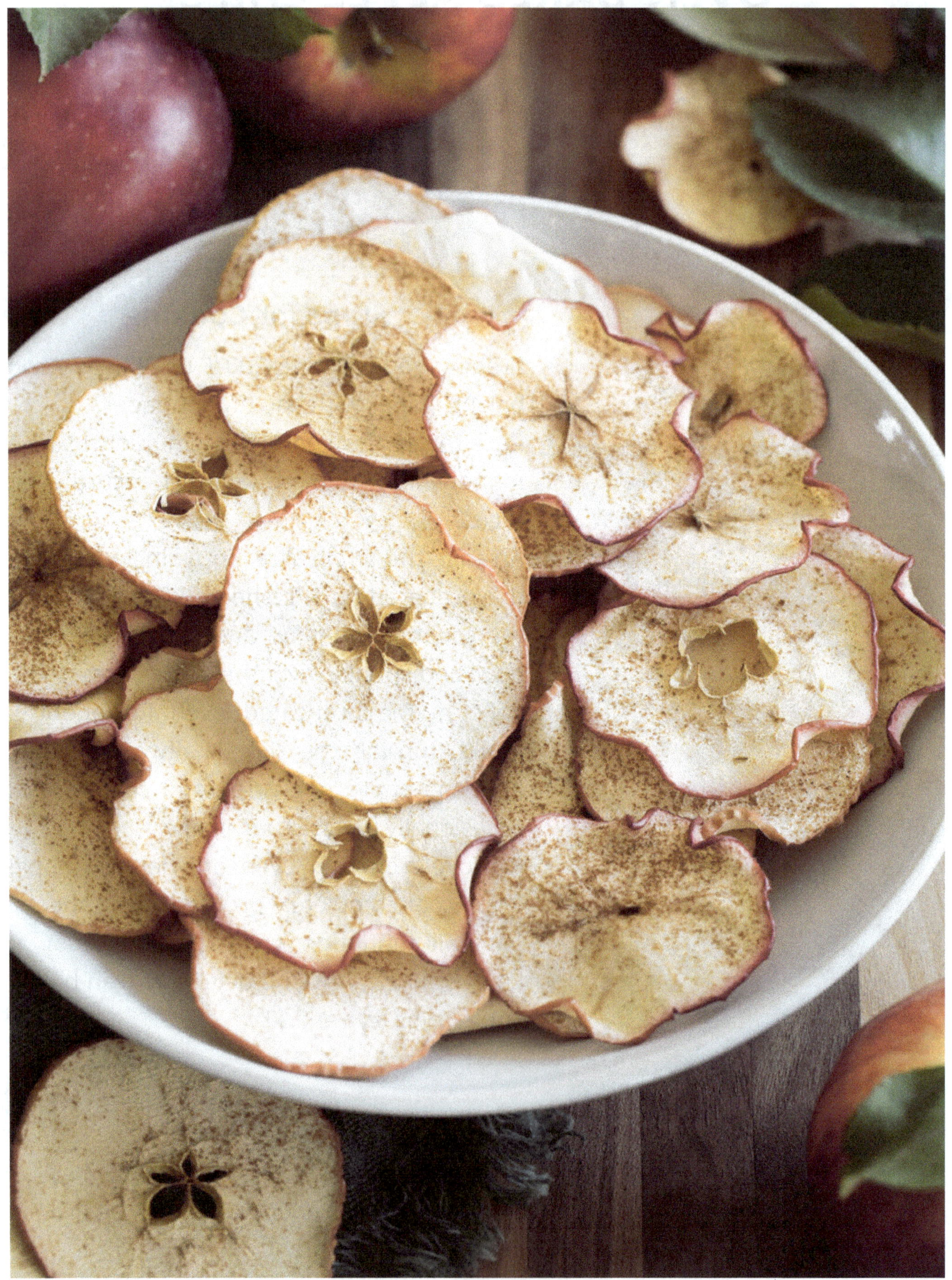

MEAL PLAN

WEEK 1

Monday
- Breakfast: Berry Smoothie
- Lunch: Spinach and Strawberry Salad
- Dinner: Baked Fish with Lemon and Herbs

Tuesday
- Breakfast: Egg and Veggie Scramble
- Lunch: Greek Salad
- Dinner: Chicken and Veggie Stir-Fry

Wednesday
- Breakfast: Fruit Salad
- Lunch: Cucumber and Tomato Salad
- Dinner: Stuffed Bell Peppers

Thursday
- Breakfast: Berry Smoothie
- Lunch: Turkey Lettuce Wraps
- Dinner: Spaghetti Squash with Marinara

Friday
- Breakfast: Egg and Veggie Scramble
- Lunch: Tomato Basil Soup
- Dinner: Shrimp and Avocado Salad

Saturday
- Breakfast: Fruit Salad
- Lunch: Zucchini Noodles with Pesto
- Dinner: Chicken and Cabbage Stir-Fry

Sunday
- Breakfast: Berry Smoothie
- Lunch: Spinach and Strawberry Salad
- Dinner: Grilled Veggie Skewers

WEEK 2

Monday
- Breakfast: Egg and Veggie Scramble
- Lunch: Broiled Grapefruit
- Dinner: Chicken Vegetable Kabobs

Tuesday
- Breakfast: Fruit Salad
- Lunch: Mango Salsa
- Dinner: Eggplant Lasagna

Wednesday
- Breakfast: Berry Smoothie
- Lunch: Grilled Pineapple
- Dinner: Chickpea Salad

Thursday
- Breakfast: Egg and Veggie Scramble
- Lunch: Roasted Carrot and Parsnip Fries
- Dinner: Quinoa and Black Bean Salad

Friday
- Breakfast: Fruit Salad
- Lunch: Stuffed Mushrooms
- Dinner: Lentil Soup

Saturday
- Breakfast: Berry Smoothie
- Lunch: Spinach and Strawberry Salad
- Dinner: Roasted Brussels Sprouts

Sunday
- Breakfast: Egg and Veggie Scramble
- Lunch: Cucumber and Tomato Salad
- Dinner: Cauliflower Fried Rice

WEEK 3

Monday
- Breakfast: Berry Smoothie
- Lunch: Shrimp and Avocado Salad
- Dinner: Chicken and Veggie Stir-Fry

Tuesday
- Breakfast: Egg and Veggie Scramble
- Lunch: Greek Salad
- Dinner: Baked Fish with Lemon and Herbs

Wednesday
- Breakfast: Fruit Salad
- Lunch: Spinach and Strawberry Salad
- Dinner: Stuffed Bell Peppers

Thursday
- Breakfast: Berry Smoothie
- Lunch: Tomato Basil Soup
- Dinner: Turkey Lettuce Wraps

Friday
- Breakfast: Egg and Veggie Scramble
- Lunch: Broiled Grapefruit
- Dinner: Chicken Vegetable Kabobs

Saturday
- Breakfast: Fruit Salad
- Lunch: Mango Salsa
- Dinner: Eggplant Lasagna

Sunday
- Breakfast: Berry Smoothie
- Lunch: Zucchini Noodles with Pesto
- Dinner: Grilled Veggie Skewers

www.ingramcontent.com/pod-product-compliance
Lightning Source LLC
Chambersburg PA
CBHW081809250726
48653CB00010B/3858